Diabetic Low-Fat
and
No-Fat Meals in Minutes

More than 250 Delicious, Easy, and Healthy
Recipes & Menus for People with Diabetes,
Their Families, and Their Friends

by

M.J. Smith, R.D.

CHRONIMED
PUBLISHING

Diabetic Low-Fat and No-Fat Meals in Minutes—More Than 250
Delicious, Easy, and Healthy Recipes & Menus for People with
Diabetes, Their Families, and Their Friends

©1996 by M.J. Smith, R.D.

Library of Congress Cataloging-in-Publication Data

M.J. Smith

Diabetic Low-Fat and No-Fat Meals in Minutes. / M.J. Smith

       p.   cm.

Includes index

ISBN 1-56561-158-6; $19.95 ($27.95 Can.)

Edited by: Jolene Steffer
Cover Design: Terry Dugan Design
Text Design: David Enyeart
Photography: John Strange Photography
Editorial Production Manager: Jeff Braun
Art/Production Manager: Claire Lewis
Printed in the United States of America

Published by
Chronimed Publishing
P.O. Box 59032
Minneapolis, MN 55459-9686

10   9   8   7   6   5   4   3   2   1

Notice

Consult Your Health Care Professional

Readers are advised to seek the guidance of a licensed physician or health care professional before making changes in health care regimens, since each individual case or need may vary. This book is intended for informational purposes only and is not for use as an alternative to appropriate medical care. While every effort has been made to ensure that the information is the most current available, new research findings, being released with increasing frequency, may invalidate some data.

Acknowledgments

Thank you to my patients and colleagues who have shared recipes and stories, and to Katie Schuster who helped with nutrient analysis.

Thank you to David Wexler at Chronimed Publishing who put his confidence in me to write this very important book, and to the Juvenile Diabetes Foundation for their partnership in sharing the low-fat/no-fat message.

Dedication

This book is written with thoughts of all the registered dietitians I know whose professional life is dedicated to helping people with diabetes... through attentive listening, creative planning, and heartfelt caring.

About the Author

Three of M.J. Smith's grandparents had insulin-dependent diabetes, so low-sugar desserts were a routine part of family holiday celebrations during her childhood. Ms. Smith began to work with people with diabetes as a dietetic extern during the summers of her college years at Allen Memorial Hospital in Waterloo, Iowa. She spent hours calculating diets, teaching the "ins and outs" of the exchange system, and helping patients fit favorite foods into their exchange prescription. Several years later in the University of Iowa Hospitals and Clinics Dietetic Internship, she mastered the Carbohydrate Counting approach and taught this method to parents and children with diabetes.

Since that time, Ms. Smith has been in dietetic practice helping people with diabetes to control their blood glucose levels. Her introductory line to clients in diet counseling is, "Do you realize that we are playing a numbers game and blood glucose control is the bottom line here?" and she follows that remark with, "My job is to teach you the 101 ways to win the numbers game with your favorite food choices."

In the 1980s, she was one of the first dietitian/authors to recognize the benefits of a low-fat diet for weight control, as well as to reduce heart disease and cancer risk. She has written seven successful low-fat cookbooks while continuing her dietetic practice. When she is not seeing patients or writing, she is in her kitchen trying new recipes, evaluating low-fat food products or working with produce from her garden.

Ms. Smith is married to Dr. Andy Smith, a family physician, and they have two school-aged children. She is a Stephen's Minister in her local church and a volunteer in her parent/teacher group. Ms. Smith is very fond of the people and lifestyle she has found in the small Mississippi River community of Guttenberg, Iowa.

Readers are encouraged to correspond with M.J. Smith by e-mail at:
mjsmithrd@worldnet.att.net

Foreword

by Jean Betschart, M.N., R.N., C.D.E

I have struggled to control my weight all my life. As a chubby child and almost obese teen, I tried to lose weight by a variety of healthy and some not-so-healthy diets. Even after I was diagnosed with diabetes, I generally tried to undercut the allowed percentage of fat in my meal plan in order to cut calories. (Not that I would recommend doing this— it is important to work with your dietitian to follow a healthy meal plan.) Eating a low-fat diet is important for people with diabetes, not only for its role in helping to prevent or delay blood vessel disease, but also for its role in preventing cancer!

My daughter, Julie, an ex-gymnast and now an exercise physiologist, is into low-fat everything. She and I have experimented, sometimes successfully but more often unsuccessfully, over the years with a multitude of recipes. She found out that if you removed the sugar, the fat and the sodium, most of what you had left was not worth eating. Between the two of us, we probably wasted more ingredients than we consumed. Son, Jeff, said he was going to create "Jeff's Soda" to accompany the low-fat, low-sodium, low-sugar delicacies we created. "Jeff's Soda" would include no artificial sugar (no real sugar), no artificial salt (no real salt), no artificial fat (no real fat), no artificial flavoring (no real flavoring) and no artificial taste (no real taste)!

However, M.J. Smith has solved the dieting dilemma. She has put together a variety of tested, delicious, practical ways to prepare recipes for people with diabetes who follow low-fat meal plans. Her other successful low-fat cookbooks have led the way to this welcome edition. She now introduces the book I wish that I had ten years ago during my "experimentation" phase. These are basic recipes that are useful to everyone, but are easy to incorporate into a diabetic meal plan, whether you use exchanges, carbohydrate counting, or another approach. They are suitable and practical for the whole family! I think you will enjoy what you find here. No longer will we have to experiment with leaving half the ingredients out while improvising on well-loved recipes. You will enjoy trying these new, creative, delicious treats from breakfast to dessert!

Jean Betschart, M.N., R.N., C.D.E.
Ms. Betschart is past president of the
American Association of Diabetes Educators
and a diabetes educator at Children's
Hospital of Pittsburgh. She is also the author
of *It's Time to Learn About Diabetes* and *A Magic Ride in Foozbah Land,* and coauthor of
In Control: A Guide for Teens with Diabetes.

Contents

Introduction

I've spent the last 15 years helping persons with diabetes understand their food choices and manage their disease; in that time I have learned two things.

First, high fat levels spell double trouble for the heart health of people with diabetes. This risk of heart disease includes microvascular (small blood vessel) complications (eye, kidney, and nerve disease) as well as large vessel, or macrovascular, disease (chest pain, heart attack, stroke, and poor circulation). For people with diabetes, three out of four hospitalizations are caused by these problems and 80 percent of people with diabetes will die of macrovascular or large vessel disease.

Abnormal levels of blood fats or lipids are partly responsible for this high risk. This low-fat/no-fat cookbook has been written to help stop the heart trouble before it starts.

A low saturated fat diet (less than 10 percent of total calories) is the best kind of nutrition insurance to prevent heart disease. When I work with young people with insulin dependent diabetes, I want them to understand that a low saturated fat diet is the answer to delaying or preventing vascular disease. And for older people with non-insulin dependent diabetes, a low-fat diet improves insulin sensitivity and function and ultimately improves blood glucose control.

A second concept that guides my diet teaching is that there are as many formulas for blood glucose control as there are persons with diabetes. Age, weight, genetics, activity pattern, exercise, fiber, fat, work schedule, frequency of illness, medications, alcohol, and gender all have something to do with how your blood glucose level behaves on any given day. Thus, it's important for persons with diabetes to have a dietitian who is a good listener to help sort this all out.

I recognize that many of our feelings about food are rooted in deep-seated emotional, family, lifestyle and cultural values. Food is literally a cultural metaphor for life. Food is often how we define ourselves in our relationships with others and it is integrally tied to nurturance, bonding and love. Our food choices are a vehicle for self affirming action and wound around individual and family values. This book will teach you to alter some of your favorite comfort foods (like Low-Fat French Toast) while building your repertoire of diabetic-friendly recipes.

Chapter One

Readings

90s-Style Diabetes Management

The Diabetes Control and Complications Trial (DCCT), which was concluded in 1993, was a multicenter, prospective, randomized clinical research study. Physicians and dietitians and nurses who study diabetes like to call this a landmark study because its results were so dramatic. This project was carefully designed to compare two types of treatment: intensive insulin therapy (frequent blood testing and frequent insulin adjustments) that aimed for achieving blood glucose levels near the nondiabetic range (< 125 mg/dl) versus conventional or standard therapy (less frequent testing and insulin adjustments). Microvascular tissues (small blood vessels) were examined before and after the study. (Note: See page 325 for more information about blood glucose levels.)

The results showed that intensive diabetes therapy results in a 50 percent overall risk reduction for diabetic microvascular complications (retinopathy and nephropathy). The blood glucose levels of the intensive therapy group averaged near 155 mg/dl, while the conventional treatment groups had blood glucose levels near 231 mg/dl. The DCCT found intensive therapy to reduce risk for onset and progression of diabetic retinopathy, kidney disease, and neuropathy. However, the tight blood sugar control achieved by intensive diabetes therapy also led to more episodes of hypoglycemia (or low blood sugar). This condition must be anticipated and treated promptly.

The study provided additional valuable information about the role of diet management including that certain individual profiles and eating habits predict a person's ability to adhere to intensive treatment plans. Researchers found that many nutrition strategies can be used to promote a consistent eating plan and that diet is the most complex aspect of diabetes therapy.

The research study made it clear to me, as a practicing dietitian, that we need to simplify and streamline nutrition priorities. Over the last 15 years I have searched in vain for a magic one-shot deal that might help everyone. Nutrition researchers have recently studied diabetic diet instruction systems (exchange system versus a simple food guide) and concluded that one type of instruction was no more effective than the other in improving glucose levels. So we're back to the idea that there are many diet prescriptions that will be successful in helping persons with diabetes control their blood glucose and blood lipids.

As you read this cookbook, you may be planning meals for a family member, or maybe you're looking for a low-sugar dessert for a visiting friend. Or perhaps you just learned that you have diabetes. As questions come to your mind, go ahead and write them down in the margin of the book. Take this along to your next visit with your physician or dietitian. Ask the health care professionals you are working with if you are being treated in accordance with the findings of the DCCT.

Back to Fats:
Sorting Out the Good from the Bad

This cookbook is a guide to reducing saturated fat in the diet with the goal of improving the heart health of people with diabetes. A recent study confirmed the importance of this goal. The Policy Analysis of Brookline, Massachusetts, studied the effect of reducing saturated fat intake on the incidence of coronary heart disease. They found 3 million first-time coronary events are estimated to occur over a 10-year period among Americans with elevated cholesterol levels. Reducing saturated fat intake by 1 to 3 percent from the current level of 9 percent would reduce heart disease by 100,000 cases by the year 2005.

A very low saturated fat intake is most helpful in reducing the bad cholesterol known as low density lipoprotein (LDL) cholesterol. Most of the cholesterol deposits in the arteries are carried by LDL.

Find out your LDL cholesterol level, and keep it under 130 mg/dl.

To reduce LDL—
    Reduce saturated fat and total fat
    Use unsaturated fats when you do use fat
    Increase fiber in the diet
    Keep blood glucose in tight control because high blood glucose
        increases LDLs in the blood.

High-density lipoproteins (HDLs) are good fats that clean cholesterol out of the circulatory system. Find out your HDL cholesterol level and keep it greater than 35 to 45 mg/dl.

To increase HDL—
    Exercise regularly
    Lose weight
    Keep blood glucose under tight control

Triglycerides are another type of fat that can be a troublemaker, increasing risk of heart disease. Find out your triglycerides level and keep it below 200 mg/dl.

To lower triglycerides—
    Reduce weight if overweight
    Exercise regularly
    Avoid alcohol
    Avoid sugar in all its forms

As you sort out the differences between good and bad fats, keep in mind that the first step you take should be to strictly limit you intake of saturated fat. Look over the following top five list to see how you are doing.

Top Five List for Limiting Saturated Fat

Do you:
1. Use the leanest possible ground meat, trim all fat (including poultry skin) from meat carefully, and limit meat portions to 2 to 3 ounces?
2. Use small amounts of very soft spreadable margarine, checking the label for the least amount of saturated fat? Do you avoid all solid fats, including stick margarine, lard, and canned shortening?
3. Use 1% or skim milk dairy products only? This includes skim or 1% fat milk, nonfat refrigerated or frozen yogurt, nonfat cream cheese, nonfat sour cream, 1% cottage cheese, and hard cheeses with less than 3 grams of fat per ounce.
4. Avoid all commercially deep-fried foods and all commercial bakery products?
5. Avoid all fatty meats, including bacon, sausage, and bologna?

If you answered yes to these five questions, you are probably doing very well in limiting saturated fat and lowering your risk of heart disease. Saturated fat may also be hiding in your diet in the form of salad dressings, snack foods, and candy.

Choosing a Food Plan
for Managing Blood Glucose

Stop on a street corner and ask five different people for directions to the nearest restaurant and you'll probably get five different answers. The same is true for the best "route" to blood sugar control. There are any number of strategies or prescriptions or plans that promote optimum blood glucose control. The following section describes the most common meal planning approaches.

Food Exchange System

The Exchange Lists for Meal Planning is a popular and useful tool to control total carbohydrates and fat. The system was developed by the American Dietetic Association and the American Diabetes Association in 1950 and has been continually updated and improved, with the latest revision coming in 1995. Foods are grouped into six lists called exchange lists. Each list is a group of measured foods of approximately the same nutrient value. Therefore, foods on each list can be substituted or "exchanged" with other foods on the same list. All of the recipes in this cookbook have been translated into food exchange values for readers using this system.

The following chart shows the amount of nutrients in one serving from each group:

	CARBOHYDRATE (G)	PROTEIN (G)	FAT (G)	CALORIES
Carbohydrate Group				
Starch	15	3	< 1	80
Fruit	15	0	0	60
Milk:				
Skim	12	8	0-3	90
Low-fat	12	8	5	120
Whole	12	8	8	150
Other carbs	15	varies	varies	varies
Vegetables	5	2	0	25
Meat and Meat Substitute Group				
Very lean	0	7	0-1	35
Lean	0	7	3	55
Medium-fat	0	7	5	75
High-fat	0	7	8	100
Fat Group	—	—	5	45

From these lists, a daily food plan is created to meet the individual's nutrient needs.

Basic Daily Food Exchange Allowances

Daily Calorie Level	1200	1400	1600	1800	2000
			Number of Exchanges		
Breakfast					
Starch	2	2	2	2	2
Fruit	1	1	2	2	2
Skim milk	1	1	1	1	1
Fat	1	1	1	1	1
Lunch					
Starch	2	2	2	2	3
Fruit	1	1	1	1	1
Skim milk	0	0	0	½	½
Lean meat	3	3	3	3	3
Vegetable	1	1	1	1	1
Fat	1	1	1	2	2
Dinner					
Starch	1	2	2	3	3
Fruit	1	1	1	1	1
Skim milk	0	0	0	½	½
Lean meat	2	2	3	3	3
Vegetable	1	2	2	2	2
Fat	0	1	1	1	1
Snack					
Starch	0	0	1	1	1
Fruit	1	1	1	1	2
Skim milk	1	1	1	1	1
Fat	0	0	0	0	1

From this basic daily prescription, a sample menu with measured foods is developed. The following is an example of an 1800 calorie meal plan using the exchange prescription.

Meal Plan for __Janet_____ Date _____6/1/96_____
Dietitian: _____M.J._____

Time	Number of Exchanges/ Choices		Menu Ideas
7AM	__5__	**Carbohydrate group**	½ cup bran flakes; 1 wheat toast; 1 cup skim milk; 8 dried apricot halves; ½ cup orange juice; 1 teaspoon soft margarine or 1 whole raisin bagel; 1 cup skim milk; 2 tablespoons reduced-fat cream cheese; 1 large banana
	__2__	**Starch**	
	__2__	**Fruit**	
	__1__	**Milk (skim)**	
	1 or 2	**Vegetables**	
	___	**Meat group**	
	__1__	**Fat group**	
12PM	__4½__	**Carbohydrate group**	2 slices rye bread; 3 ounces lean turkey; lettuce, pickles, sprouts; 1 cup cantaloupe; ½ cup skim milk; 2 teaspoons soft margarine or 1 whole toasted English muffin; ¾ cup cottage cheese; 3 tablespoons wheat germ; ½ cup pineapple tidbits; ½ cup tomato juice; 2 teaspoons soft margarine; ½ cup skim milk
	__2__	**Starch**	
	__1__	**Fruit**	
	__½__	**Milk (skim)**	
	__3__	**Meat group (lean)**	
	__2__	**Fat group**	
3PM	__1__	fruit	1¼ cup strawberries or 1¼ cup watermelon
	___	___	
6PM	__6½__	**Carbohydrate group**	1 small baked potato; 1 dinner roll; 3 ounces broiled salmon; 1 cup steamed broccoli; ½ cup skim milk; 1 cup raspberries; 1 teaspoon tartar sauce or 1 hamburger roll; 3 ounces lean hamburger; ½ large pear; 6 soda crackers; 1 cup vegetable broth; ½ cup skim milk; 1 tablespoon low-fat mayonnaise
	__3__	**Starch**	
	__1__	**Fruit**	
	__½__	**Milk (skim)**	
	1 or 2	**Vegetables**	
	__3__	**Meat group (lean)**	
	__1__	**Fat group**	
8PM	__1__	skim milk	1 cup skim milk and ¼ cup low-fat granola or 1 cup fruited yogurt without sugar and 8 animal crackers
	__1__	starch	

	Grams	Percent
Carbohydrate	230	51%
Protein	112	24%
Fat	48	25%
Calories	1800	100%

The advantage of the Food Exchange System is that it promotes careful control of calories, carbohydrates, protein, and fat. When medicine and/or insulin is used to control blood glucose, the exchange system is a good companion that allows for a consistent, moderate, low-fat food intake. However, for some individuals, the concept of "exchanging" foods is difficult to understand. In addition, common food labels and home-style recipes may be difficult to translate into food exchanges.

No-Concentrated-Sweets Diet

The No-Concentrated-Sweets Diet is a black and white, yes or no approach to blood glucose control. This is a list of foods allowed and foods to avoid to control blood glucose. Low-sugar, low-fat substitutions are recommended. All of the recipes in this cookbook are allowed on the No-Concentrated-Sweets Diet. A sample of this diet follows.

Food Group	*Foods to Limit*	*Substitutions*
Breads, Cereals, Rice and Pasta (6-11 servings/day) • 1 slice of bread • 1 oz. of cereal • 1 tortilla • 1/2 c. rice or pasta • 3 c. popcorn • 4 plain crackers	Sweetened cereals Most pastries and donuts Frosted bread items Regular muffins and quick breads Granola Bars	Unsweetened cereals Use bagels or English muffins Plain cinnamon rolls Low sugar quick breads (1/4 c. sugar per loaf or per doz. muffins)
Vegetables (3-5 servings/day) • 1 c. of raw leafy vegetables • 1/2 c. of other vegetables	Vegetable salads with sugar Sweet pickled foods Sweet and sour salads	Use sugar substitute in dressings
Fruit (2-4 servings/day) • 1 medium apple, banana, orange, nectarine, or peach • 1/2 c. of chopped, cooked or canned fruit	Fruit packed in syrup Fruit drinks Frozen fruit w/ sugar Fruit roll-ups	Juice-packed fruits 100% fruit juice Frozen whole fruits Fresh fruit or dried fruit

Food Group	*Foods to Limit*	*Substitutions*
• 3/4 c. of fruit juice • 1/4c. of dried fruit		
Milk, Yogurt, and Cheese (2-3 servings/day) • 1 c. of 1% or skim milk or yogurt • 1 1/2 oz. of reduced fat cheese (< 3 g. fat/ounce)	Sugar-sweetened yogurts Ice cream, ice milk, sherbet, and frozen yogurt Hot cocoa mixes Pudding mixes	Sugar-free yogurt Sugar-free frozen desserts Sugar-free cocoa mixes Sugar-free pudding mixes Choose reduced-fat cheeses
Meats, Poultry, Fish, Dry Beans, Eggs (2-3 servings/day) • 2-3 oz. of cooked lean meat, poultry, or fish • 1 oz. of meat = 1/2c. of cooked dry beans, 1 egg, or 2 T. peanut butter	All fried meats All poultry skin Fatty meats such as corned beef, regular pastrami, short ribs, spareribs, rib eye cuts, fatty ground beef, hot dogs, bacon and regular luncheon meats. Limit eggs to 4 per week.	Bake, broil, grill, roast or steam meats. Look for very lean ground beef or drain and rinse ground beef. (1 cup very hot water per pound of browned meat. Allow to drain 5 minutes.) Use low-fat luncheon meats
Sugars and Sweets • Choose sugar substitutes only	Sugar at the table or in cooking Honey, brown and powdered sugar Corn and maple syrup, fructose Jam, jelly, and apple butter	Sugar substitutes such as Equal, Sweet'n Low Sweet 10, Weight Watchers or Sweet 1 Sugar-free jams or fruit spreads
Added Fats • 1-2 tsp. added fat per meal	Deep fried foods Whipped toppings Sweet salad dressings such as French and Western Butter, stick margarines, peanut butter, canned shortenings	Choose 1000 Island, Ranch, Italian dressings Choose a soft margarine made from liquid oil such as corn, soy, canola, or olive Choose light mayonnaise

Food Group	Foods to Limit	Substitutions
Others	Soft drinks	Sugar-free soft drinks
	Candy and gum	Sugar-free mints and
	Cakes	gum
	Cookies and bars	Angel food cake (for
	Cheesecakes, pies	special occasions)
	Refrigerated desserts	Low sugar recipes for
	Gelatin mixes	cookies
	Alcoholic beverages	Sugar-free dessert
		mixes
		Limit to 1 serving
		with food in accor-
		dance with physician's
		advice. (12 oz. beer, 5
		oz. wine, or 1 1/2 oz.
		liquor)

The advantage of the No-Concentrated-Sweets Diet is that it does not involve counting calories, carbohydrates, or food exchanges. It is used most successfully by the normal weight person with diabetes who has an acute sense of fullness and does not abuse portions of carbohydrate-containing foods. The disadvantage is that the diet allows no method for the occasional inclusion of sugar containing foods.

Carbohydrate Counting

Carbohydrate counting is based on the assumption that carbohydrate intake is the main consideration in determining meal-related insulin requirements, while protein and fat may be less important. There is an identifiable ratio between the number of grams of carbohydrate a person eats and the number of units of insulin he or she needs to utilize them. This ratio also varies greatly among persons with diabetes, from as little as 5 grams of carbohydrate per unit of insulin to as many as 20 grams. A general rule of thumb is that lower ratios are typical in insulin-resistant individuals with non-insulin dependent diabetes and higher ratios are seen in lean, fit persons with insulin-dependent diabetes.

The process of counting grams of carbohydrate is simple. All of the recipes in this cookbook include the carbohydrate count. Food counting books provide carbohydrate counts, and most food labels state the number of grams of carbohydrate per serving. One of my favorite references is *The Complete Book of Food Counts* by Corinne T. Netzer. Write to Dell Readers Service, Box DR, 1540 Broadway, New York, NY 10036, to order the book. Carbohydrate counting is used most successfully by people with diabetes who have mastered insulin adjustment and insulin supplementation prior to learning carbohydrate counting and who are seeking flexibility in meal planning, while maintaining blood glucose control. This approach requires a commitment to daily recording of food intake, activity and blood glucose testing; and to frequent interaction with a dietitian or diabetes team. Here is an example of Daily Carbohydrate Counting:

Breakfast/morning snack Quota: 60–65 grams	Actual
8 ounces nonfat sugar-free cherry yogurt	15
1/3 cup lowfat granola	15
1/2 cup orange juice	15
Tea	0
1/2 wheat bagel	15
1 tablespoon lowfat cream cheese	5
Total	**60**

Lunch/ afternoon snack Quota: 70–75 grams	Actual
3 ounces lean smoked turkey	0
leaf lettuce, mustard, chopped tomato	0
1/2 pita bread (check label)	20
1 large pear	20
1 cup chocolate skim milk (check label)	25
1 1/2 cups popcorn	7
Diet Coke	0
Total	**72**

Dinner/evening snack Quota: 70–75 grams	Actual
2 slices Hand Tossed Veggie Lover's Pizza	56
Large fresh vegetable salad	5
2 tablespoons lowfat Italian Dressing	0
1 cup skim milk	12
Herbal mint tea	0
Total	**73**

To explore carbohydrate counting further, order *Carbohydrate Counting: Getting Started* from The American Dietetic Association by calling 800-877-1600, ext. 5000. (Catalog no. 6003; cost is less than $10.)

The disadvantage of this system is that carbohydrate counting does not promote a varied intake of grains, cereals, fruits, vegetables, and skim milk products. Instead, these foods are all thrown together for a simple carbohydrate count. A cornerstone of optimal nutrition is a varied diet.

The Food Guide Pyramid

The Food Guide Pyramid is a popular illustration of foods to eat. The pyramid promotes the use of grains, fruits, and vegetables to form the base of the diet. As the Pyramid ascends to the peak, less emphasis is placed on high-fat, high-sugar foods.

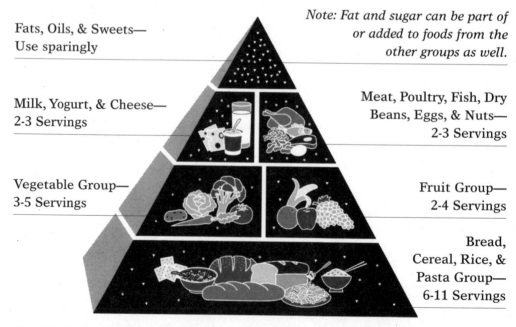

Fats, Oils, & Sweets—
Use sparingly

Note: Fat and sugar can be part of or added to foods from the other groups as well.

Milk, Yogurt, & Cheese—
2-3 Servings

Meat, Poultry, Fish, Dry Beans, Eggs, & Nuts—
2-3 Servings

Vegetable Group—
3-5 Servings

Fruit Group—
2-4 Servings

Bread, Cereal, Rice, & Pasta Group—
6-11 Servings

The Food Guide Pyramid may be used successfully by persons with diabetes to promote blood glucose control. Reducing fats, oils, and sweets (as well as fat-containing meats, cheeses, and dairy products), while increasing fat-free grains, fruits, and vegetables may be the single most effective dietary prescription for persons with diabetes. The recipes in this book fit the pyramid.

Safe Use of Sweeteners

The concept that sugar is forbidden for persons with diabetes is well understood. To review this in the most basic of terms: If a person lacks insulin action to transport sugar (or glucose) out of the blood to the cells where it can be utilized, then sugar is best avoided. Sugar is not essential to a nutrient-rich diet, as it contains no vitamins, minerals, or protein. There are also many forms of sugar to avoid that go by other names, including brown sugar, corn syrup, dextrose, fructose, glucose, honey, lactose, maltose, mannitol, sorbitol, xylitol, maple sugar, and molasses.

But humans are born with a preference for the sweet taste. Restricting your sugar intake requires planning ahead and food and recipe experimentation along with blood glucose monitoring. Recent research has shown that if blood glucose is in good control and triglycerides (blood fats) are within normal range, a small amount of sugar (1 teaspoon in a meal) may not cause a problematic rise in blood glucose.

Persons with diabetes have three options for dealing with sweeteners:
   a. You can avoid all forms of sugar and sugar substitutes and adapt the taste buds to the natural sweetness from fruits and sweet spices such as nutmeg, cinnamon, vanilla, or almond. (See recipe for Apple Cinnamon Pull Apart Buns for an example.)
   b. You can avoid all forms of sugar, enjoy sweetness from fruits and spices, and carefully use sugar substitutes to replace the sugar. I have tested several common sugar substitutes in these recipes to demonstrate their individual usefulness. (See Sugar Twin in Banana Nut Crunch Muffins, see Equal Measure in Chocolate Almond Mousse, see Sweet One in Pumpkin Custard.) You'll want to experiment with your own favorite sugar substitutes; examples are shown on the following page.

The chart below compares common sugar substitutes:

Generic Name	Fructose	Saccharin	Aspartame	Acesulfame K
Trade Name	Estee SweetLite Sucaryl Zero-Cal Superose	Sugar Twin Sweet'n Low Spoonfuls NatraTaste	Equal Sweetmate	Sweet One Estee SwissSweet
Sugar Equivalent	Fructose (Powder)	Saccharin (Powder)	Equal (Packets)	Sweet One (Packets)
2 tsp.	2/3 tsp.	1/5 tsp.	1 packet	1 packet
1 Tbsp.	1 tsp.	1/3 tsp.	1 1/2 packets	1 1/4 packets
1/4 cup	4 tsp.	3 packets	6 packets	3 packets
1/3 cup	5 1/3 tsp.	4 packets	8 packets	4 packets
1/2 cup	8 tsp.	6 packets	12 packets	6 packets
2/3 cup	3 1/2 Tbsp.	8 packets	16 packets	8 packets
3/4 cup	1/4 cup	9 packets	18 packets	9 packets
1 cup	1/3 cup	12 packets	24 packets	12 packets

These sugar substitutes have an appropriate role within the context of a healthy diet and are best used in moderation and with the approval of your physician.

c. The third option is to enjoy the sweetness of fruits and spices, carefully use sugar substitutes, and experiment with small amounts of sugar in the diet. For instance, most recipes for quick-breads can be adapted to 1/4 cup of sugar per loaf or 1/4 cup of sugar per dozen muffins. In cake recipes, the sugar can be reduced by one third or one half (use 2/3 cup or 1/2 cup instead of 1 cup) without changing the taste and texture (see recipe for Morning Glory Muffins as an example). Many recipes in this book include directions for using a small amount of sugar or a sugar substitute (see Fluffy Fruit Dip).

50 Ways to Do Without Sugar and Fat with Herbs, Spices, and Seasonings

Now that we have cut sugar and fat from the diet, it's time to add back some flavor. If you don't have many herbs, spices, and seasonings in your cupboard, consider this your invitation to a whole new world of cooking. There is some evidence that spices and herbs can stimulate the potency of insulin. Dr. Richard Anderson at USDA tested sage, oregano, turmeric, cloves and cinnamon and found them to boost insulin activity. Look over this list and remember, these are just some ideas to get you started. Your favorite tricks with herbs and spices will be those you discover yourself.

1. Mix equal parts of basil, dill weed, garlic, and parsley and use instead of cheese or meat in an omelet.

2. Mix one part oregano, two parts marjoram, and three parts sage to season poultry dishes.

3. For Italian flavor, mix equal parts basil, marjoram, oregano, rosemary, sage, savory, and thyme and use with plain tomato sauce and pasta.

4. For a barbecue flavor, mix cumin, garlic, hot pepper, and oregano. Rub into lean meat before grilling.

5. Keep a combination of basil, parsley, and savory in a shaker container for seasoning cooked vegetables.

6. Add rosemary to plain old chicken noodle soup.

7. Enjoy the flavor of tarragon in turkey vegetable soup.

8. Rub pork chops with ginger and thyme before baking.

9. Use dried mint as a rub for lamb chops.

10. Add dill weed to salmon loaf.

11. Sprinkle oregano on your low-fat toasted cheese sandwich.

12. Chives give a mild onion flavor to cottage cheese.

13. Use dill seed on green beans.

14. Sprinkle nutmeg and cinnamon on cream of wheat cereal.

15. Add 1/4 teaspoon almond flavoring to sugar-free low-fat cocoa.

16. Mix 1 teaspoon maple flavoring into your pancake batter.

17. Spice up a three bean salad with fennel.

18. Add chopped fresh cilantro to any Mexican dish.

19. Guarantee premium flavor by crushing whole spices with a mortar and pestle just before use.

20. Whenever possible, choose fresh parsley, basil, and chives over dried herbs.

21. Use a kitchen shears or sharp knife to cut the leaves of fresh herbs very finely to release maximum flavor.

22. A good rule of thumb is that 1/4 teaspoon of powdered herbs is equivalent to 3/4 to 1 teaspoon of dried flaked herbs or 2 teaspoons of fresh herbs.

23. When adding spices and herbs to cold recipes, allow the food to refrigerate at least 2 hours for the flavors to blend.

24. Add fresh spices and herbs to hot dishes as close to serving time as possible for the most flavorful results.

25. Dried herbs and spices should be added early in the cooking process to prevent a powdery taste.

26. Release dried herb flavor by browning the herbs in a skillet that has been sprayed with nonstick cooking spray. Then combine with meat or vegetables.

27. Fresh herbs are most flavorful just before the plant flowers.

28. Store herbs in a cool dry place with minimum exposure to air and sunlight.

29. Bunches of fresh herbs can be tied together at the stem and dried upside down in a cool place for a week.

30. You can also use the microwave oven to dry fresh herbs. Place the clean dry leaves in a single layer between two paper towels and microwave on high for 2 to 2 1/2 minutes.

31. Fresh herbs can be washed and sealed in freezer bags in small quantities or chopped and frozen in water in ice cube trays for use in sauces or soups.

32. Give ordinary turkey and noodles an Indian flavor by adding 1/2 to 1 teaspoon of dried curry powder.

33. Try a combination of allspice and cloves on your oatmeal instead of sugar.

34. Sprinkle your waffles with cardamom and cinnamon and top with sugar-free nonfat vanilla yogurt.

35. Sprinkle a little basil on your fresh sliced summer tomatoes and say good-bye to sugar and salt.

36. Grate some fresh cinnamon stick on your grapefruit.

37. If you're doing without salt, bay leaves are a must in soups and stews.

38. Caraway seed is a wonderful complement to low-fat cabbage salad or slaw.

39. Low-fat potato salad is spiced up with celery seed.

40. Chervil is a sweet herb with a very delicate flavor most loved in marinated vegetable salads.

41. Juniper berries reduce the wild flavor in venison and wild game.

42. Mace is an English spice suitable for a low-sugar pumpkin pie.

43. Marjoram is closely related to oregano, but it's a bit more delicate and flowery.

44. Don't forget fruit rinds when it comes to intensifying flavor. Finely grated orange, lemon, tangerine, or lime zest can save a low-sugar dessert.

45. Paprika is best added just before serving or it may turn brown.

46. Poppy seeds make any rice dish more fun.

47. Use sage, dill, anise, and fennel in salads to accompany bean and legume dishes as they are thought to help prevent intestinal gas.

48. Spice up your lunch with chili pepper if you feel a cold coming on. Hot foods thin secretions in the air passages. If you eat hot food, not only do your eyes water, but so do your lungs.

49. For the best quality mail order herbs, spices, and seasoning blends, call Penzeys, Ltd., at 414-574-0277 or write P.O. Box 1448, Waukesha, WI 53187.

50. If you want more information about herbs, be sure to pick up the authoritative guide to herbs called *Magic Herbs.* It's available from Chronimed Publishing at 1-800-848-2793.

Friendly Fiber—An Aid to Blood Glucose Control

While diabetic diets strictly limit saturated fat and sugar, the opposite is true of dietary fiber. Fiber, that part of grains, legumes, vegetables, fruits, seeds, and skins that is not digested by the body is of great help in controlling blood glucose. Fiber seems to stop or slow the rise in blood glucose after meals. A high fiber meal also promotes a feeling of fullness, as digestive activity continues longer than without a fiber component.

Top 10 Ways to a High Fiber Diet Every Day

1. Include a raw vegetable at both lunch and dinner.

2. Include a raw fruit at one snack time. The best choices are fresh apples, pears, and peaches with the skins left on or berries of any kind.

3. Get into the habit of eating a high fiber cereal for breakfast or before bed.

4. Include dried beans and peas, lima beans, or lentils at least twice a week.

5. Use 100 percent whole wheat or cracked wheat bread.

6. Always eat the skin from a potato.

7. Start buying brown rice instead of white.

8. Use wheat buns, bagels, and English muffins instead of white.

9. Substitute wheat pilaf, couscous, or bulgur for plain white pasta.

10. Keep dried apricots or prunes in the car and cupboard as a quick way to stave off hunger.

Counting Fiber Grams

The American Cancer Society recommends 30 grams of fiber daily. Use the chart below to check your diet. Dietary-Fiber Content of Common Foods has been researched by Dr. James D. Anderson, Professor of Medicine and Clinical Nutrition at the University of Kentucky. If you are interested in obtaining further information about the High Fiber Diet for Diabetes, write to him in care of HCF Nutrition Research Foundation, Box 22124, Lexington, Kentucky 40522.

Dietary-Fiber Content of Common Foods

Grams of Dietary Fiber
(rounded to nearest whole number)

Fruits

Apple, 1 small with skin, 3 gm.
Applesauce, canned, unsweetened, 1/2 cup, 2 gm.
Apricots, canned, drained, 4 halves, 1 gm.
Apricots, dried, 7 halves, 2 gm.
Avocado, fresh, 1/8, 1 gm.
Banana, fresh, 1 small, 2 gm.
Blackberries, fresh, 3/4 cup, 4 gm.
Blueberries, fresh, 3/4 cup, 1 gm.
Cherries, fresh, black, 12 large, 1 gm.
Cherries, red, canned, 1/2 cup, 2 gm.
Cranberries, fresh, 1/2 cup, 2 gm.
Currants, fresh, 1 cup, 4 gm.
Dates, dried, 2 1/2 medium, 1 gm.
Figs, dried, 1 1/2, 2 gm.
Figs, fresh, 2, 3 gm.
Fruit cocktail, canned, 1/2 cup, 2 gm.
Gooseberries, fresh, 3/4 cup, 3 gm.
Grapefruit, canned, 1/2 cup, 1 gm.
Grapefruit, fresh, 1/2 medium, 2 gm.

Grams of Dietary Fiber
(rounded to nearest whole number)

Grapes, fresh, red, with skin, 15 small, <1 gm.
Grapes, fresh, white, with skin, 15 small, 1 gm.
Guava, fresh, 1, 5 gm.
Kiwi fruit, 1 large, 2 gm.
Mango, fresh, 1/2 small, 3 gm.
Melon (cantaloupe, honeydew, or watermelon), 1 cup cubed, 1 gm.
Nectarine, fresh, 1, 2 gm.
Orange, fresh, navel, 1 small, 2 gm.
Orange, fresh, others, 1 small, 3 gm.
Orange, mandarin, canned, 3/4 cup, 1 gm.
Orange juice, 1/2 cup, 1 gm.
Peaches, canned, 1/2 cup, 2 gm.
Peaches, dried, 1/6 cup (2 2/3 tablespoons), 2 gm.
Peaches, fresh, 1 medium, 2 gm.
Pears, canned, 1/2 cup, 4 gm.
Pears, fresh, 1 small, 3 gm.
Pineapple, canned, 1/2 cup, 2 gm.
Pineapple, fresh, 3/4 cup, 1 gm.
Plums, greengage, fresh, 2 medium, 3 gm.
Plums, purple, canned, 1/2 cup, 3 gm.
Plums, fresh, 2 medium red, 2 gm.
Pomegranate, fresh, inc. seeds & juice, 1/2, 3 gm.
Prunes, dried, 3 medium, 2 gm.
Raisins, dried, 2 tablespoons, <1 gm.
Raspberries, canned, 1/2 cup, 4 gm.
Raspberries, fresh, 1 cup, 3 gm.
Rhubarb, fresh, 2 cups, 4 gm.
Strawberries, fresh, 1 cup, 2 gm.

Vegetables

Asparagus, cooked, 1/2 cup, 2 gm.
Asparagus, canned, 1/2 cup, 3 gm.
Bean sprouts, fresh, 1 cup, 2 gm.
Beets, canned or cooked fresh, 1/2 cup, 2 gm.

Grams of Dietary Fiber
(rounded to nearest whole number)

Broccoli, cooked, 1/2 cup, 2 gm.
Brussel sprouts, cooked, 1/2 cup, 4 gm.
Cabbage, fresh, 1 cup, 2 gm.
Cabbage, red, cooked, 1/2 cup, 3 gm.
Cabbage, red, fresh, 1 cup, 3 gm.
Carrots, canned, or sliced, cooked, 1/2 cup, 2 gm.
Carrots. fresh, 1 7 1/2" long, 2 gm.
Cauliflower, fresh, cooked, 1/2 cup, 1 gm.
Cauliflower, fresh, 1 cup, 2 gm.
Celery, fresh, chopped, 1 cup, 2 gm.
Corn, canned, whole kernel, 1/2 cup, 2 gm.
Corn on the cob, cooked, 6" ear, 2 gm.
Cucumber, fresh, sliced, 1 cup, 1 gm.
Eggplant, cooked, 1/2 cup, 1 gm.
Endive, fresh, 1 cup, 1 gm.
Green beans, cooked, 1/2 cup, 2 gm.
Green beans, French cut, cooked, 1/2 cup, 3 gm.
Kale, chopped, frozen, 1/2 cup, 3 gm.
Leeks, sliced, cooked, 1/2 cup, 1 gm.
Lettuce, 1 cup, 1 gm.
Mushrooms, fresh, 1 cup pieces, 1 gm.
Okra, fresh, trimmed pods, 1 cup slices, 7 gm.
Olives, canned, 10 small, 1 gm.
Onions, fresh or cooked, chopped, 1/2 cup, 2 gm.
Parsley, fresh, 1 tablespoon, 1 gm.
Peas, green, canned, 1/2 cup, 3 gm.
Peas, green, fresh, cooked, 1/2 cup, 2 gm.
Peas, green, frozen, cooked, 1/2 cup, 4 gm.
Peppers, green, fresh, chopped, 1 cup, 2 gm.
Potatoes, sweet, canned, 1/3 cup, 1 gm.
Potatoes, sweet, cooked, 1/3 cup, 3 gm.
Potatoes, white, fresh with skin, 1/2 cup, 2 gm.
Pumpkin, fresh, cooked, 1 cup, 1 gm.
Radish, fresh, 1 cup slices, 1 gm.

Grams of Dietary Fiber
(rounded to nearest whole number)

Snow peas, fresh, microwaved, 1/2 cup, 1 gm.
Spinach, cooked, fresh or frozen, 1/2 cup, 2 gm.
Squash, yellow crookneck, frozen, 1/2 cup, 1 gm.
Tomatoes, canned, 1/2 cup, 1 gm.
Tomato, fresh, 1 medium, 1 gm.
Tomato sauce, 1/3 cup, 1 gm.
Turnips cooked, 1/2 cup, 5 gm.
Watercress, fresh, 1 cup, 1 gm.
Yams, cooked, 1/3 cup, 1 gm.
Zucchini, fresh, 1 cup, 2 gm.
Zucchini, sliced, cooked, 1/2 cup, 1 gm.

Legumes

Black beans, cooked, 1/2 cup, 6 gm.
Black-eyed peas, canned, 1/2 cup, 5 gm.
Broad beans, cooked, 1/2 cup, 5 gm.
Butter beans, dried, cooked, 1/2 cup, 7 gm.
Chick peas, dried, cooked, 1/2 cup, 4 gm.
Cranberry beans, dried, cooked, 1/2 cup, 5 gm.
Garbanzo beans, canned, 1/3 cup, 3 gm.
Kidney beans, dark red, cooked, 1/2 cup, 7 gm.
Kidney beans, light red, canned, 1/2 cup, 8 gm.
Lentils, dried, cooked, 1/2 cup, 5 gm.
Lentils, red, dried, cooked, 1/2 cup, 2 gm.
Lima beans, canned, 1/2 cup, 4 gm.
Mung beans, dried, cooked, 1/2 cup, 3 gm.
Navy beans, dried, cooked, 1/2 cup, 7 gm.
Pinto beans, canned or dried, cooked, 1/2 cup, 6 gm.
Pork and beans with sauce, canned, 1/2 cup, 5 gm.
Split peas, dried, cooked, 1/2 cup, 3 gm.
White beans, Great Northern, canned, 1/2 cup, 7 gm.
White beans, Great Northern, dried, cooked, 1/2 cup, 5 gm.

Nuts and Seeds

Almonds, 6 whole, 1 gm.

Grams of Dietary Fiber
(rounded to nearest whole number)

Brazil nuts, 1 tablespoon, 1 gm.
Chestnuts, microwaved, 2 tablespoons, 1 gm.
Coconut, dried, 1/2 tablespoon, 2 gm.
Coconut, fresh, 2 tablespoons, 1 gm.
Hazelnuts (filberts), 1 tablespoon, 1 gm.
Peanut butter, smooth, 1 tablespoon, 1 gm.
Peanuts, fresh or roasted, 10 large, 1 gm.
Sesame seeds, 1 tablespoon, 1 gm.
Sunflower seeds, 1 tablespoon, 1 gm.
Walnuts, 6 whole, 1 gm.

Cereals

Kellogg's All Bran, 1/3 cup, 9 gm.
Kellogg's All Bran with Extra Fiber, 1/2 cup, 14 gm.
General Mills Cheerios, 1 1/4 cups, 3 gm.
Kellogg's Cornflakes, 1 cup, 1 gm.
Cream of Wheat, regular, uncooked, 2 1/2 tablespoons, 1 gm.
General Mills Fiber One, 1/2 cup, 12 gm.
40% Bran Flakes, 2/3 cup, 4 gm.
Post Grape Nuts, 1/4 cup, 3 gm.
Grits, corn, quick, uncooked, 3 tablespoons, 1 gm.
Kellogg's Nutri-Grain Wheat, 2/3 cup, 3 gm.
Quaker Oat Bran, cooked, 3/4 cup, 4 gm.
Oat Bran, uncooked, 1/3 cup, 4 gm.
Raisin Bran, 3/4 cup, 5 gm.
Shredded Wheat, 2/3 cup, 4 gm.
Kellogg's Special K, 1 cup, 1 gm.
Bran Buds, 1 cup, 23 gm.
100% Bran, 1 cup, 20 gm.
Oatmeal, cooked, 1 cup, 2 gm.
Rolled Wheat, cooked, 1 cup, 8 gm.
Cornmeal, 1 cup, 3 gm.
Popcorn, popped, 3 cups, 2 gm.

Grams of Dietary Fiber
(rounded to nearest whole number)

Flours

All-purpose, 1 cup, 4 gm.
Bread and cake, 1 cup, 4 gm.
Rye, 1 cup, 18 gm.
Whole wheat, 1 cup, 15 gm.
Oat, 1 cup, 12 gm.

Starches

Barley, pearl, uncooked, 2 tablespoons, 3 gm.
Macaroni, white, cooked, 1/2 cup, 1 gm.
Macaroni, whole wheat, cooked, 1/2 cup, 2 gm.
Noodles, egg or spinach, cooked, 1/2 cup, 1 gm.
Rice, brown, or white, cooked, 1/2 cup, 1 gm.
Spaghetti, white, cooked, 1/2 cup, 1 gm.
Spaghetti, whole wheat, cooked, 1/2 cup, 3 gm.
Wheat bran, 1/2 cup, 12 gm.
Wheat germ, 3 tablespoons, 4 gm.

Breads and Crackers

Bagel, plain, 1 bagel, 1 gm.
Bread, bran, cracked wheat, rye, whole wheat, mixed grain, 1 slice, 2 gm.
Bread, oatmeal, raisin, sourdough, white, pita, French, 1 slice, 1 gm.
Bread, pumpernickel, 1 slice, 3 gm.
Bread, mixed grain, wheat or white "lite," 1 slice, 6 gm.
Bread sticks, 2, 1 gm.
Bun, hamburger, 1, 1 gm.
Cornbread, 2" cube, 1 gm.
Crackers, 6 saltine, 5 saltine wheat, 5 white melba toast, 1 gm.
Crackers, 2 graham squares, 3 gm.
English muffin, 1 whole, 2 gm.
Pretzels, hard, 3/4 ounce, 1 gm.
Roll, 1 brown and serve, 1 French, 1 gm.
Tortilla, 1 flour or corn or 1 taco shell, 1 gm.

Does Your Picky Eater Have Diabetes?

If you are caring for a child with diabetes who also happens to be a fussy eater, you have a double challenge to meet. All children learn early in life that the dinner table is a perfect place to assert independence. Parents are concerned that children get enough to eat at meals, and children often use this concern to ensure that they are served only the foods they want to eat.

Mealtime can become a battle of wills. If these battles are not diffused, children may never accept a balanced and varied diet that provides optimum nutrition from the basic food groups. This is especially true for children with diabetes.

How do we convince children of the importance of good nutrition?

Preschool children can be told that they need food to grow and be healthy. You can share more details as children reach school age with comments such as, "Food has things in it called nutrients. These nutrients are vitamins, minerals, protein, fat, carbohydrates, and water that are essential as our body grows."

Use concrete comparisons and examples. "See how big you are now compared to when you were a baby? Your body uses the nutrients in food to help you grow.

"Your body uses nutrients to maintain its defense system against colds, flu, and sicknesses. Vitamins, minerals, and nutrients are needed by your body to build bones, tissues, and blood. Your body uses all the different nutrients in food for energy so you can run fast, jump high, and learn quickly. If you don't get enough of the energy nutrients, you will be too tired to do your best."

Emphasize the concept that because certain foods are highly nutritious, they should be eaten more often that other nutrient-poor foods. Fruits are a good choice because they are good sources of beta carotene, vitamin C and fiber.

Children are suspicious of new foods; this fear is perfectly normal. Children are born with "uneducated" palates and need encouragement to experiment with new tastes.

Introducing new foods can be easy. Simply look at the hundreds of food options available. The goal is to have children readily accept a variety of food and vegetable tastes. With each step you take to broaden food preferences, be careful not to pass on your own dislikes. It is common for there to be one or two items that every person, parent and child alike, will not eat or drink.

Children, if left to their own devices, will eat the right amount of food to maintain their individual growth schedules, even if that amount varies greatly from day to day. It is more important that children consume quality foods, those high in essential nutrients, rather than specific quantities of food.

Parents need to accept the fact that deciding how much their children eat is a shared responsibility. Children have as much say in what they will or will not eat as you have. You can teach the importance of good nutrition with your example and by keeping an inventory of nutritious choices in the house, but we must trust children to do their part.

Raw vegetables are often more appealing to children than cooked vegetables. The flavors created by cooking some vegetables are often too strong for children. A child may have to taste a new food up to a dozen times before accepting it. Ask them to smell it the first time, taste a bite the second time, and work their way up from there.

Top 10 Ways to Cope with Picky Eaters

1. Introduce new foods at the beginning of meals, when children are most hungry and willing to try at least one bite.

2. Present new items in small portions that aren't overwhelming.

3. If children have a negative reaction to a new food before or after tasting it, remove the item from the table without comment or debate.

4. Don't give up on foods that have been rejected. Items children turn down one day might be better received a few days later.

5. Be creative in the way new foods are presented on plates. Make designs with the placement of foods or serve vegetables that are cut into geometric shapes.

6. Don't bribe or reward children for trying new foods. They must learn to like the food for its taste, not for what they receive by eating it.

7. Introduce new foods in an enthusiastic manner, selling children on the appeal of the food.

8. Set a good example by tasting new foods and showing that you enjoy trying new things.

9. Consider serving at least one brightly colored item with each meal— try an orange slice, red pepper slices, or melon balls.

10. Think variety when shopping and cooking, aiming to introduce one out-of-the-ordinary food every week.

6 Weeks of Diabetic Low-Fat/ No-Fat Menus

A series of daily menu ideas is provided on the following pages to help you put it all together. The menus are designed to provide less than 25 percent of calories from fat and less than 10 percent of calories from saturated fat. They are high in fiber and include three meals plus a snack every day. The menus can be used just as they are written and will fit with your instruction system, whether you are using the No-Concentrated-Sweets Diet, the Food Guide Pyramid, Carbohydrate Counting or the Exchange Lists. What you need to do is to write in the portion size of each menu item, depending on what your individual prescription for carbohydrates, exchanges, or food groups is.

In all likelihood, the menus will just give you a place to get started. We all get tired of the "same old thing" and often need a booster shot to get us out of our tired old meal patterns. There are ideas for big weekend breakfasts, brown bag lunches, fast food and carryout meals, Saturday Nights out and daily snacks.

Recipes for the italicized items are included in this book.

Breakfast	*Lunch*	*Dinner*

Week One

Sunday

Orange juice	*Clam Chowder*	*Pink Slush*
Low-Fat French Toast	Breadsticks	Pizza with
Soft margarine	*Spinach Salad with*	veggie toppings
All-fruit spread	*Canadian Bacon*	*Waldorf Salad*
Skim milk	Soft margarine	*Oatmeal Raisin Cookie*
	Kiwi Frozen Treat	Skim milk
	Hot tea	

Snack: Reduced-fat microwave popcorn

Monday

Fresh grapefruit sections	Lean turkey with	Show-off Tamale Pie
Flaked cereal	fresh sprouts and	Lettuce, tomato, and
Apple Oatbran Muffin	mustard on an	fresh peppers on the side
Soft margarine	onion bagel	*Banana Pudding*
Skim milk	Fresh apple	Skim milk
	Oatmeal Raisin Cookie	
	Mineral water	

Snack: *Party Hearty Cereal Mix*

Tuesday

Pineapple juice	Leftover Tamale Pie	*Bean and Bacon*
Crunchy Pita Breakfast	Baby carrots with	*Casserole*
Skim milk	reduced-fat dressing dip	Corn bread muffins
	Green grapes	Fresh salad with
	Iced tea	reduced-fat dressing
		Leftover Banana Pudding
		Skim milk

Snack: Low-fat sugar-free cocoa

Breakfast	Lunch	Dinner

Wednesday

Breakfast	Lunch	Dinner
Hot oatmeal with	Vegetable soup	*Nonfat Fried Chicken*
dried pineapple tidbits	Low-fat	Baked potato
Raisin toast	cottage cheese	Nonfat sour cream
Soft margarine	Fresh peach slices	*Coconut Cole Slaw*
Skim milk	Reduced-fat	Reduced-fat, sugar-free
	wheat crackers	frozen yogurt
	Sugar-free soft drink	Skim milk

Snack: Frozen fruit cups

Thursday

Grape juice	Leftover chicken on	*Orange and Spice*
Bran cereal	wheat bread with	*Grilled Pork*
Fresh raspberries	spicy mustard, lettuce,	*Scalloped Corn*
English muffin	and pickles	Celery sticks
Soft margarine	Reduced-fat potato chips	Hot applesauce
Skim milk	Pear slices	over nonfat,
	Herb tea	sugar-free yogurt
		Skim milk

Snack: *Low-fat Ranch dip with veggies*

Friday

Sliced fresh orange	FAST FOOD LUNCH	Tomato juice
Toasted blueberry bagel	Baked potato with	*Muffin-sized*
Soft margarine	chili topping	*Meatloaves*
All-fruit spread	Green salad with	*Mushroom Risotto*
Skim milk	reduced-fat salad dressing	*Frosted*
	Orange juice	*Raspberry Salad*
		Skim milk

Snack: Reduced-fat soft cheese with pretzel dippers

Breakfast	Lunch	Dinner

Saturday

Breakfast	Lunch	Dinner
Hot apple cider	*Paella Shrimp*	SATURDAY NIGHT OUT!
Skinny Quiche Lorraine	*Salad*	Stuffed mushrooms
Wheat toast	Broiled french bread	Fresh green salad
Soft margarine	Soft margarine	with reduced-fat
All-fruit spread	Sliced watermelon	dressing
Skim milk	*Kahlua Mousse*	Dinner roll
		Petite cut sirloin
		Rice pilaf
		Decaf coffee

Week Two

Sunday

Breakfast	Lunch	Dinner
Orange juice	*Gazpacho*	*Sangria*
Low-fat Pancakes	Breadsticks	Tacos with beans and
Soft margarine	*Salmon Pasta Salad*	reduced-fat cheese
All-fruit spread	Soft margarine	*Pineapple Lover's*
Skim milk	*Peach Pie*	*Salad*
	Hot tea	*Date Bar*
		Skim milk

Snack: Fat-free, sugar-free frozen fudge bar

Monday

Breakfast	Lunch	Dinner
Fresh grapefruit sections	Lean ham with	*Chicken Creole*
Flaked cereal	fresh sprouts and	Lettuce, tomato,
Golden Morning Muffins	mustard on an	and fresh peppers
Soft margarine	onion bagel	on the side
Skim milk	Fresh apple	*Strawberry Dessert*
	Date Bar	*Soufflé*
	Mineral water	Skim milk

Snack: *Crispix Mix*

	Breakfast	Lunch	Dinner

Tuesday

Breakfast	Lunch	Dinner
Pineapple juice	Leftover Chicken Creole	*Shepherd's Pie*
German Fruit Bread	Baby carrots with	Fresh green salad
Nonfat cream cheese	reduced-fat salad	with reduced-fat
All-fruit preserves	dressing dip	salad dressing
Skim milk	Fresh nectarine	Leftover Strawberry
	Iced tea	Dessert
		Skim milk

Snack: *Fluffy Fruit Dip* with apple slices

Wednesday

Breakfast	Lunch	Dinner
Hot oatmeal with	Chicken-noodle soup	*Double Orange*
golden raisins	Low-fat string cheese	*Roughy*
Cracked wheat toast	Italian breadsticks	*Old-fashioned*
Soft margarine	Fresh pear slices	*Fried Potatoes*
Skim milk	Sugar-free soft drink	*Copper Penny*
		Salad
		Reduced-fat,
		sugar-free ice milk
		Skim milk

Snack: *Banana Spread* with a half bagel

Thursday

Breakfast	Lunch	Dinner
Grape juice	Water-pack tuna	*Peach Slush*
Bran cereal	and nonfat mayonnaise	*Chinese Pork*
Fresh blueberries	on a bun with	*with Bamboo Shoots*
Hawaiian Bread	lettuce and pickles	Steamed rice
in the Machine	Reduced-fat	*Almond Custard*
Soft margarine	potato chips	Skim milk
Skim milk	Fresh apricot	
	Herb tea	

Snack: Sugar-free lemon yogurt

Breakfast	Lunch	Dinner

Friday

Sliced fresh orange	FAST FOOD LUNCH	Tomato juice
Toasted raisin bagel	Grilled chicken on a	*Corned Beef & Kraut*
Soft margarine	bun with lettuce	*in the Crockpot*
All-fruit spread	and pickles	Mashed potatoes
Skim milk	Green salad with	*Diet Mt. Dew Salad*
	reduced-fat salad	Skim milk
	dressing	
	Orange juice	

Snack: *Let the Good Times Roll Cheeseball*

Saturday

Hot cranberry juice	*Lemon Chicken*	SATURDAY NIGHT OUT!
Scrambled Eggs	*Salad*	Shrimp cocktail
and Cheese	Broiled french bread	Coleslaw
Wheat toast	Soft margarine	Dinner roll
Soft margarine	Sliced watermelon	Broiled pork chop
All-fruit spread	*Chocolate Almond Mousse*	Baked potato
Skim milk	Decaf coffee	Decaf coffee

Week Three

Sunday

Orange juice	*Black Bean Soup*	*Five-minute Roast*
Apple Cinnamon	Broiled flour tortilla	*Beef 'n Salsa*
Pull Apart Rolls	with reduced-fat	*Sandwiches*
Soft margarine	cheddar cheese	*Creamy Nonfat*
Skim milk	*Raspberry Cream*	*Coleslaw*
	Cheese Dessert	Skim milk
	Hot tea	

Snack: Reduced-fat microwave popcorn

Breakfast	Lunch	Dinner

Monday

Fresh grapefruit sections	Lean turkey with fresh sprouts and mustard on an onion bagel	*Layered Italian Zucchini Casserole*
Flaked cereal		French bread
Carrot Bread in the Machine	Fresh apple	Soft margarine
Soft margarine	Baby carrots	Sliced cucumbers with reduced-fat ranch dressing
Skim milk	Mineral water	*Apple Crunch*
		Skim milk

Snack: Fruited yogurt

Tuesday

Pineapple juice	Leftover zucchini casserole	*Red Beans and Rice*
Pear and Lemon Bread in the Machine	Baby carrots with reduced-fat salad dressing dip	Cornbread muffins
Skim milk		Fresh green salad with reduced-fat salad dressing
	Red grapes	*Peppermint Pears*
	Iced tea	Skim milk

Snack: Low-fat, sugar-free cocoa

Wednesday

Hot oatmeal with dried apricots	Chicken and Rice Soup	*Scalloped Kabobs*
Raisin toast	Low-fat string cheese	Baked potato
Soft margarine	Fresh peach slices	Nonfat sour cream
Skim milk	Reduced-fat wheat crackers	*Jicama and Fruit Salad*
	Iced tea	Skim milk

Snack: *Frozen Fruit Cups*

Breakfast	*Lunch*	*Dinner*

Thursday

Grape juice	Turkey on wheat bread	*Baked Ham with*
Bran cereal	with spicy mustard,	*Pear Glaze*
Fresh raspberries	lettuce, and pickles	Mashed potatoes
English muffin	Reduced-fat	*Sweet and Sour*
Soft magarine	potato chips	*Three Bean Salad*
Skim milk	Pear slices	Fresh raspberries
	Herb tea	Skim milk

Snack: *Blender Eggnog*

Friday

Sliced fresh orange	FAST FOOD LUNCH	*Indian Chicken in*
Toasted wheat bagel	Baked potato	*the Crockpot*
Soft margarine	with cheese and	Steamed rice
All-fruit spread	broccoli topping	*One-bowl Lemon-*
Skim milk	Green salad with	*Dressed Fruit Salad*
	reduced-fat salad	Skim milk
	dressing	
	Orange juice	

Snack: Sugar-free ice milk

Saturday

Hot apple cider	*Ham and Cheddar*	SATURDAY NIGHT OUT!
Poppy Seed Surprise	*Chef Salad*	Marinated
Flaked cereal	Broiled french bread	artichoke hearts
Soft margarine	Soft margarine	Fresh green salad
Skim milk	Sliced watermelon	with reduced-fat
	Cappuccino Parfait	dressing
		Dinner roll
		Grilled tuna
		Rice pilaf
		Decaf coffee

Breakfast	Lunch	Dinner

Week Four

Sunday

Breakfast	Lunch	Dinner
Orange juice	Pineapple-orange	*Crunchy Beef Burritos*
Pumpkin Nut Bread	juice	Lettuce, tomatoes, and
in the Machine	*Fish & Mixed*	nonfat sour cream
Nonfat cream cheese	*Vegetable Stew*	*Everyone's Favorite*
Skim milk	Breadsticks	*Strawberry Pie*
	Lemon Angel Cookies	Skim milk

Snack: Reduced-fat microwave popcorn

Monday

Breakfast	Lunch	Dinner
Fresh grapefruit sections	Lean roast beef	*Chicken à la King*
Flaked cereal	with fresh sprouts	Fresh greens with
Pineapple Bran Muffin	and catsup on an	*Caesar Salad Dressing*
Soft margarine	onion bagel	Sugar-free chocolate
Skim milk	Fresh peach	pudding with sliced
	Leftover lemon cookie	bananas
	Mineral water	Skim milk

Snack: Fat-free pretzels

Tuesday

Breakfast	Lunch	Dinner
Pineapple juice	Leftover Chicken	*Pepsi and Pork*
Banana Nut	à la King	*in the Crockpot*
Crunch Muffin	Baby carrots with	Steamed bowtie pasta
Cream of wheat	reduced-fat salad	with reduced-fat
Skim milk	dressing dip	margarine
	Red grapes	Fresh green salad with
	Iced tea	reduced-fat salad dressing
		Fruit cocktail
		Skim milk

Snack: Low-fat, sugar-free cocoa

Breakfast	Lunch	Dinner

Wednesday

Hot oatmeal with dried pineapple tidbits Raisin toast Soft margarine Skim milk	Tomato soup Low-fat cottage cheese Fresh pear slices Reduced-fat wheat crackers Sugar-free soft drink	*Salmon Loaf* Baked potato Nonfat sour cream *Creamy Cucumber Salad* Reduced-fat, sugar-free frozen yogurt Skim milk

Snack: *Orange Fruit Sicle*

Thursday

Grape juice Bran cereal Fresh strawberries English muffin Soft margarine Skim milk	Reduced-fat peanut butter with all-fruit spread on wheat bread Tomato juice Pineapple spears Herb tea	*One-Dish Oven Beef Stew* Buttermilk biscuits *Sugar-free Perfection Salad* Hot applesauce over nonfat, sugar-free frozen yogurt Skim milk

Snack: *Chocolate Strawberries*

Friday

Sliced fresh orange Toasted honey whole-grain bagel Soft margarine All-fruit spread Skim milk	FAST FOOD LUNCH Lean roast beef sandwich with taco sauce Green salad with reduced-fat salad dressing Orange juice	FRIDAY NIGHT OUT! Vegetable soup Fresh spinach salad with reduced-fat dressing Hard roll Broiled turkey breast with mustard sauce Baked potato Decaf coffee

Breakfast	*Lunch*	*Dinner*

Saturday

Hot apple cider	*Pork and Brown Rice*	Cornflake Chicken
Poached egg	*Salad*	*Potato Casserole*
Low-fat Sausage Patties	Broiled french bread	*in the Microwave*
Wheat toast	Soft margarine	Steamed broccoli
Soft margarine	*Minted Honeydew*	and carrots
Skim milk	*Melon*	Cantaloupe
	Mineral water	Skim milk

Snack: *Creamy Cherry Pie*

Week Five

Sunday

Orange juice	*Hamburger*	Pineapple-grapefruit
Low-fat Pancake	*Vegetable Soup*	juice
Soft margarine	*Green Chili Bread*	*Sloppy Joe Pizza*
All-fruit spread	Reduced-fat margarine	Lettuce on the side
Skim milk	*Apple Pie*	Skim milk
	Hot tea	

Snack: Fat-free, sugar-free frozen fudge bar

Monday

Fresh grapefruit	Lean ham with fresh	Vegetable juice
Flaked cereal	sprouts and mustard	*Chicken Pot Pie*
Pineapple Orange	on an onion bagel	Wheat roll with
Bread in the Machine	Fresh apple	reduced-fat margarine
Soft margarine	*Chewy Double*	*Citrus Salad*
Skim milk	*Chocolate Cookies*	Skim milk
	Mineral water	

Snack: *Crispix Mix*

Breakfast	*Lunch*	*Dinner*

Tuesday

Pineapple juice	Leftover chicken	*Sausage-Stuffed Peppers*
Cranberry Lemon Bread	pot pie	Kaiser roll
in the Machine	Baby carrots with	Fresh green salad
Soft margarine	reduced-fat salad	with reduced-fat
Skim milk	dressing dip	salad dressing
	Fresh nectarine	Leftover chocolate
	Iced tea	cookies
		Skim milk

Snack: *Fluffy Fruit Dip* with apple slices

Wednesday

Hot oatmeal with	Reduced-fat cream of	*Seafood and*
golden raisins	mushroom soup	*Asparagus Stirfry*
Cracked wheat toast	Low-fat cheddar cheese	Steamed rice
Soft margarine	Wheat crackers	Reduced-fat, sugar-
Skim milk	Fresh pear slices	free ice milk
	Sugar-free soft drink	Skim milk

Snack: *Banana Spread* with a half bagel

Thursday

Grape juice	Water-pack tuna and	*Grilled Italian*
Bran cereal	nonfat mayonnaise	*Steak Sandwich*
Fresh blueberries	with lettuce,	*Pea Salad*
Maple Date	tomato, and pickles	Sliced honeydew
Pecan Bread	Reduced-fat	melon
Soft margarine	potato chips	Skim milk
Skim milk	Fresh apricot	
	Herb tea	

Snack: Sugar-free lemon yogurt

Breakfast	*Lunch*	*Dinner*

Friday

Sliced fresh orange	FAST FOOD LUNCH	FRIDAY NIGHT OUT!
Toasted raisin bagel	Grilled chicken with	Veggie pizza
Soft margarine	lettuce and pickles	Baby carrots
All-fruit spread	Green salad with	*Five-Minute*
Skim milk	reduced-fat dressing	*Five-Cup Salad*
	Orange juice	Sugar-free cola

Snack: *Creamy Cherry Pie*

Saturday

Hot cranberry juice	*Long-Cook Bean*	SATURDAY NIGHT OUT!
Poached egg	*and Ham Soup*	Shrimp cocktail
Wheat toast	Broiled french bread	Green salad with
Soft margarine	Soft margarine	reduced-fat dressing
All-fruit spread	*Orange Pineapple Salad*	Dinner roll
Skim milk	Mineral water	Petite cut prime rib
		Baked potato
		Soft margarine
		Decaf coffee

Week Six

Sunday

Orange juice	Pineapple-orange juice	Grilled chicken on
Sunshine Muffins	*Red Beans and Rice*	a bun with lettuce,
Nonfat cream cheese	*in One Skillet*	tomato, and pickles
Skim milk	Reduced-fat	*15-Minute Potluck*
	taco chips	*Vegetable Salad*
	Sugar-free lemon yogurt	Fresh strawberries
		over sugar-free
		ice milk
		Skim milk

Snack: Reduced-fat microwave popcorn

Breakfast	Lunch	Dinner

Monday

Fresh grapefruit sections	Lean roast beef	*Stove-top Turkey*
Flaked cereal	with fresh sprouts	*and Noodles*
Wheat toast	and catsup on an	*Fat-free Creamy*
Soft margarine	onion bagel	*Italian Salad Dressing*
All-fruit spread	Reduced-fat	over greens
Skim milk	taco chips	Sugar-free vanilla
	Fresh peach	pudding with
	Mineral water	mandarin oranges
		Skim milk

Snack: Fat-free pretzels

Tuesday

Pineapple juice	Leftover turkey	*Slow-Cook Pork*
Cracked Wheat Bread	and noodles	*Picnic Pasta Salad*
in the Machine	Baby carrots with	Fruit cocktail
Soft margarine	reduced-fat salad	Skim milk
Cream of wheat	dressing dip	
Skim milk	Tangerine	
	Iced tea	

Snack: Low-fat, sugar-free cocoa

Wednesday

Hot oatmeal with	Tomato soup	*Salmon Patties*
dried pineapple tidbits	Low-fat cottage	*Fat-free Tartar Sauce*
Raisin toast	cheese	Baked potato
Soft margarine	Fresh pear slices	Nonfat sour cream
Skim milk	Reduced-fat wheat	*Tangy Marinated*
	crackers	*Onion Salad*
	Sugar-free soft drink	Reduced-fat, sugar-
		free frozen yogurt
		Skim milk

Snack: *Orange Fruit Sicle*

Breakfast	Lunch	Dinner

Thursday

Grape juice	Reduced-fat peanut	*Broccoli, Ham, and*
Bran cereal	butter and all-fruit	*Potato Casserole*
Fresh strawberries	spread on whole	Buttermilk biscuits
English muffins	wheat bread	Celery sticks
Soft margarine	Tomato juice	Sugar-free cherry
Skim milk	Pineapple spears	gelatin with sugar-
	Herb tea	free applesauce
		Skim milk

Snack: Pineapple spears

Friday

Sliced fresh orange	FAST FOOD LUNCH	FRIDAY NIGHT OUT!
Toasted honey whole	Lean roast beef	Green salad with
grain muffin	sandwich on a bun	reduced-fat dressing
Soft margarine	with taco sauce	Spaghetti with veggies
Skim milk	Green salad with	and tomato sauce
	reduced-fat dressing	Parmesan cheese
	Orange juice	on the side
		French bread
		Sugar-free soft drink

Saturday

Hot cranberry juice	*Tex-Mex Salad*	Tangerine-orange juice
Toaster waffles	White dinner roll	*Broiled Salmon*
All-fruit spread	Soft margarine	*with Chives*
Soft margarine	Watermelon	*Low-fat Potato Salad*
Skim milk	Mineral water	Steamed green beans
		Sugar-free chocolate
		ice milk
		Skim milk

Snack: *Cappuccino without the Machine*

Chapter Two

Beverages, Appetizers, *and* Snacks

Antipasto Dip for Breadsticks

Preparation time: 15 minutes
Chilling time: 30 minutes

8 servings—1/4 cup each

1/2 cup reduced-fat mayonnaise
1/2 cup nonfat sour cream
4-ounce jar artichoke hearts, drained and chopped
1/2 cup chopped roasted red peppers or 2 tablespoons
   dried red peppers
1/4 teaspoon minced garlic
1 teaspoon dried basil
1/4 teaspoon dried oregano

1. In a mixing bowl, combine all ingredients. Cover and chill at least
30 minutes to combine flavors. Serve with Italian breadsticks.

50 calories per serving
2 gm. fat, 2 gm. protein, 9 gm. carbohydrate,
0 cholesterol, 206 mg. sodium.

For exchange diets, count: 2 vegetables.

Asparagus Guacamole

Preparation time: 15 minutes

8 servings—1/3 cup each

10-ounce package frozen cut asparagus
1/4 cup nonfat mayonnaise or salad dressing
1/2 teaspoon minced garlic
2 teaspoons lime juice
2 tablespoons green chilies, drained and chopped
1/8 teaspoon salt
1/4 teaspoon cumin
1/8 teaspoon white pepper
1 green onion, chopped fine
1 small tomato, chopped fine

1. Cook asparagus according to package directions. Drain well and pat dry with a paper towel. Place asparagus in a blender container. Add next 7 ingredients, and process until smooth. Fold in chopped onion and tomato, and transfer to a serving bowl. Serve with reduced-fat tortilla chips such as Highland Northern Lights.

20 calories per serving
0 fat, 1 gm. protein, 4 gm. carbohydrate,
0 cholesterol, 144 mg. sodium.

For exchange diets, count: 1 vegetable.

Bagel Pizza

After-school treats never tasted so good!
And your kids will still be hungry for supper.

Preparation time: 10 minutes
Broiling time: 3 minutes

4 servings—1/2 bagel each

2 plain bagels, sliced in half
1/2 cup your favorite spaghetti sauce
2 ounces part-skim mozzarella cheese, shredded

1. Slice bagels in half and place on a baking sheet. Spread sauce on bagels and sprinkle with cheese. Broil 4 to 5 inches away from a low flame for 3 minutes. Open the oven door and watch as cheese melts and browns. Remove pizzas from the oven and serve.

183 calories per serving
5 gm. fat, 9 gm. protein, 25 gm. carbohydrate,
10 mg. cholesterol, 400 mg. sodium.

For exchange diets, count: 1 starch, 1 lean meat, 1 fat.

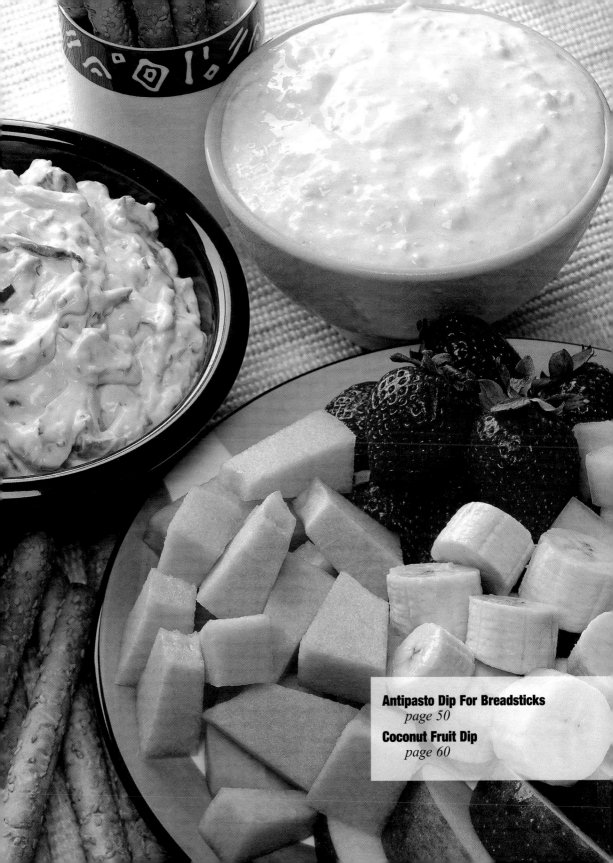

Antipasto Dip For Breadsticks
page 50

Coconut Fruit Dip
page 60

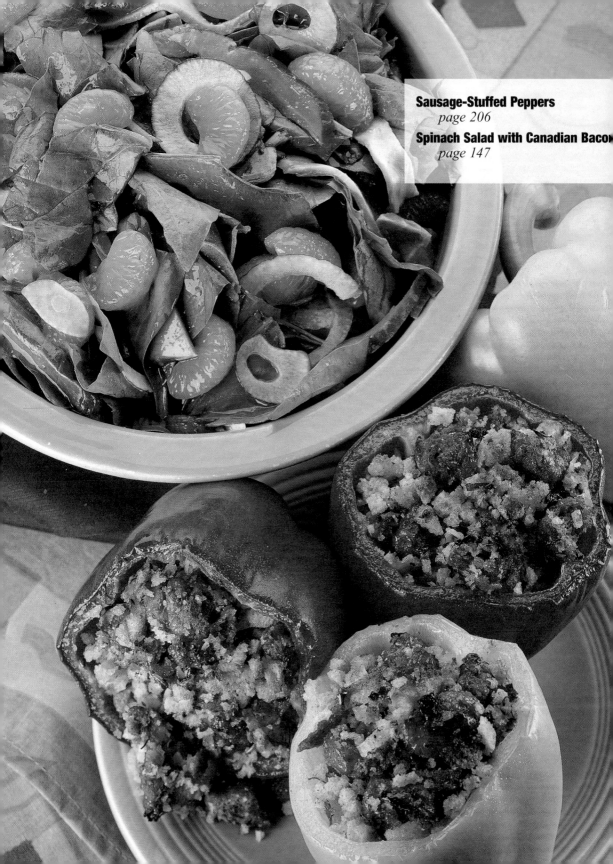

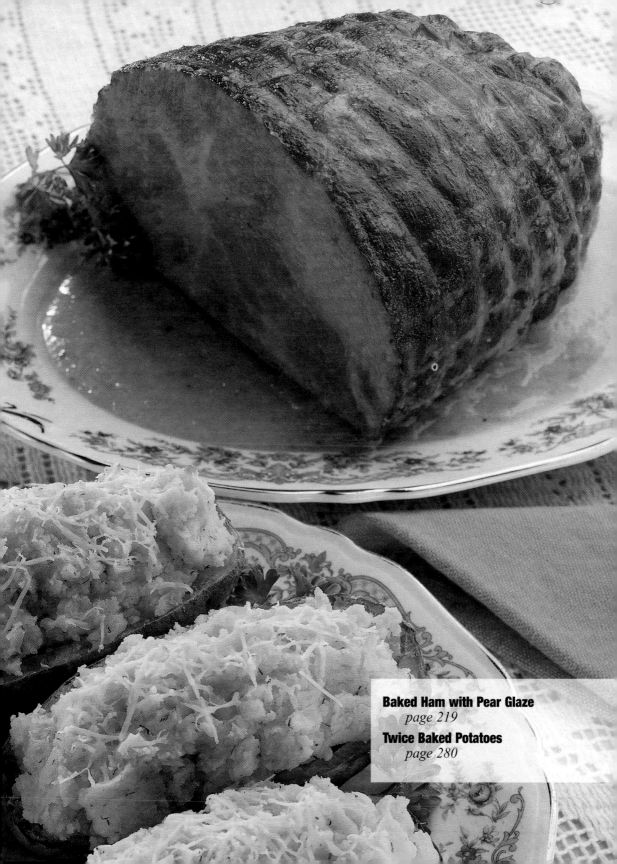

Baked Ham with Pear Glaze
page 219

Twice Baked Potatoes
page 280

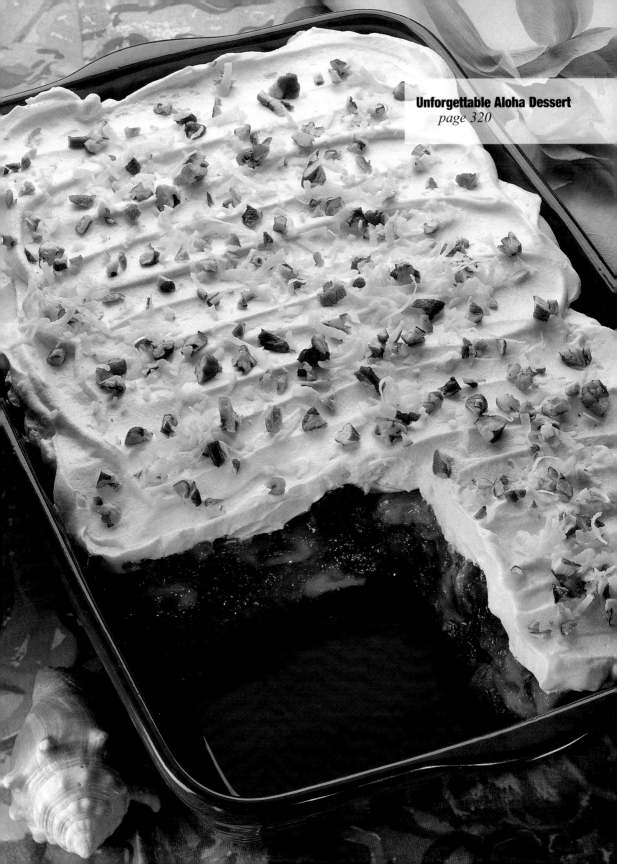

Unforgettable Aloha Dessert
page 320

Bagels with Fruit and Cheese

Preparation time: 10 minutes

8 servings—1/2 bagel each

4 plain bagels
1/2 cup nonfat ricotta cheese
1/2 cup all-fruit preserves

1. Slice bagels in half and toast until crispy.

2. Mix fruit preserves with ricotta cheese and spread over toasted bagels.

153 calories per serving
1 gm. fat, 4 gm. protein, 31 gm. carbohydrate,
3 mg. cholesterol, 238 mg. sodium.

For exchange diets, count: 1 starch, 1 fruit.

Banana Spread for Bagels

Preparation time: 15 minutes

8 servings—1/4 cup each

8 ounces reduced-fat cream cheese, softened
4 ripe bananas, mashed
fresh squeezed juice from 1/2 lemon

1. Combine all ingredients in a small bowl. Refrigerate in a covered container, and use with honey whole grain bagels. This may be used immediately or refrigerated for up to 3 days.

71 calories per serving
0 fat, 4 gm. protein, 14 gm. carbohydrate,
1 mg. cholesterol, 83 mg. sodium.

For exchange diets, count: 1 fruit.

Blender Egg Nog

Preparation time: 15 minutes

8 servings—4 ounces each

1 cup nonfat dry milk
1/2 cup Equal Measure sugar substitute
2 cups skim milk
1/2 cup water
2 whole eggs or 1/2 cup liquid egg substitute
1 teaspoon rum extract
garnish: nutmeg

1. Combine first four ingredients in a blender container, and process on high power for 3 minutes until smooth and creamy. Add eggs or substitute and rum extract; blend on low for 1 more minute. Pour into 8 short, squat cups, and garnish with nutmeg.

67 calories per serving
0 fat, 7 gm. protein, 8 gm. carbohydrate,
3 mg. cholesterol, 106 mg. sodium.

For exchange diets, count: 1/2 skim milk, 1 very lean meat.

Blue Cheese Seafood Dip

Preparation time: 15 minutes
Chilling time: 30 minutes

8 servings—6 ounces each

1 tablespoon finely grated lemon peel
3 ounces reduced-fat cream cheese, softened
7-ounce can water-packed tuna, crab or salmon,
    drained well and flaked
1/3 cup crumbled blue cheese
1 whole green onion, diced fine

1. Combine all ingredients in a small mixing bowl, and stir to blend well. Refrigerate at least 30 minutes. Serve with breadsticks or toasted pita bread triangles.

81 calories per serving
3 gm. fat, 10 gm. protein, 2 gm. carbohydrate,
18 mg. cholesterol, 273 mg. sodium.

For exchange diets, count: 2 very lean meat.

Cappuccino Without the Machine

Preparation time: 10 minutes

4 servings—6 ounces each

1 cup evaporated skim milk
1 tablespoon sugar or Nutrasweet Spoonful
    sugar substitute
2 cups strong freshly brewed coffee
sprinkle of cinnamon

1. Place milk in a 2-cup glass measuring cup. Microwave on high for 1 minute.

2. Place hot milk and sugar or sugar substitute in a blender container. Cover with a vented lid and blend until frothy, about 1 minute.

3. To serve, divide coffee into 4 mugs. Top each with frothy milk and a sprinkle of cinnamon.

58 calories per serving (47 calories with sugar substitute)
0 fat, 4 gm. protein, 10 gm. carbohydrate,
(7 gm. carbohydrate with sugar substitute),
2 mg. cholesterol, 68 mg. sodium.

For exchange diets, count: 1 fruit.
(Count 1/2 skim milk with sugar substitute.)

Cheese Nachos

After school or after work, these take the edge off hunger.

Preparation time: 10 minutes
Broiling time: 6 minutes
4 servings—1 tortilla each

4 ounces reduced-fat cheddar cheese, shredded
4 6-inch flour tortillas
1/4 cup chopped green chilies

1. Sprinkle cheddar cheese on tortillas. Top with diced green chilies. Then place on a baking sheet, and broil under low heat until crispy, about 4 to 6 minutes.

160 calories per serving
5 gm. fat, 5 gm. protein, 22 gm. carbohydrate,
20 mg. cholesterol, 276 mg. sodium.

For exchange diets, count: 1/2 skim milk, 1/2 fat, 1 starch.

Cinnamon Spread for Bagels

Preparation time: 10 minutes

8 servings—1/4 cup each

8 ounces fat-free cream cheese, softened
1 teaspoon cinnamon
1/2 cup chopped golden raisins

1. Combine all ingredients in a small bowl. Refrigerate in a covered container, and use with whole wheat bagels. This may be served immediately or kept in the refrigerator for 1 week.

50 calories per serving
0 fat, 3 gm. protein, 9 gm. carbohydrate,
1 mg. cholesterol, 84 mg. sodium.

For exchange diets, count: 1/2 skim milk.

Coconut Fruit Dip

Preparation time: 15 minutes
Chilling time: 2 hours

12 servings—1/4 cup each

8-ounce package reduced-fat cream cheese,
   softened to room temperature
1/4 cup dried coconut
1 tablespoon finely grated lemon rind
   (lime or tangerine also work well)
1 cup sugar-free vanilla refrigerated yogurt
1 teaspoon vanilla extract
1/3 cup Equal Measure sugar substitute

1. Combine ingredients in a mixing bowl and stir to mix. Chill at least 2 hours before serving with assorted fresh fruit dippers.

51 calories per serving
2 gm. fat, 3 gm. protein, 4 gm. carbohydrate,
1 mg. cholesterol, 71 mg. sodium.

For exchange diets, count: 1/2 skim milk.

Cran-Raspberry Finger Gelatin

Preparation time: 15 minutes
Chilling time: 4 hours

24 servings—1 square each

4 envelopes Knox unflavored gelatin
3 (3-ounce) packages sugar-free raspberry gelatin (may
    substitute orange gelatin)
4 cups low-calorie cranberry juice cocktail, brought to
    a boil (use orange juice with orange gelatin)

1. In a large bowl, combine Knox gelatin and flavored gelatin. Add boiling fruit juice, then pour into an 11" x 7" shallow dish. Chill for at least 4 hours. Cut into small cubes.

8 calories per serving
0 fat, 0 protein, 2 gm. carbohydrate,
0 cholesterol, 2 mg. sodium.

For exchange diets, count: as a free food.

Creamy Egg Nog

Preparation time: 15 minutes

8 servings—4 ounces each

6 eggs, separated, or 2 cups liquid egg substitute and
  6 egg whites
2 tablespoons sugar or 2 tablespoons Nutrasweet
  Spoonful sugar substitute
2 cups skim milk
2 teaspoons rum flavoring
garnish: nutmeg

1. In a large mixing bowl, beat the yolks or egg substitute well, then gradually beat in the sugar. Pour in milk slowly, beating constantly. Add the rum flavoring.

2. In a medium-size mixing bowl, beat egg whites until stiff; carefully fold into egg mixture. Fill cups and garnish with nutmeg.

103 calories per serving (90 calories with sugar substitute)
2 gm. fat, 12 gm. protein, 7 gm. carbohydrate (4 gm. carbohydrate with
sugar substitute), 161 mg. cholesterol with eggs,
(2 mg. cholesterol with egg substitute), 184 mg. sodium.

For exchange diets, count: 1/2 skim milk, 1 lean meat.
(Count 1 skim milk with sugar substitute.)

Crispix Mix

Preparation time: 15 minutes
Baking time: 1 hour

20 servings—1/2 cup each

8 cups Crispix cereal
1 cup reduced-fat peanuts (such as Planters)
1 cup mini knot pretzels
3 tablespoons reduced-fat margarine, melted
1/4 teaspoon garlic salt
1/4 teaspoon onion salt
2 teaspoons lemon juice
4 teaspoons Worcestershire sauce

1. Preheat oven to 250°.

2. Combine cereal, nuts, and pretzels in a 13" x 9" baking pan, and set aside.

3. Melt margarine in a 1 cup glass measure. Stir in all remaining ingredients and then pour over cereal, gently stirring until cereal is evenly coated. Bake for 1 hour, stirring every 15 minutes. Cool to room temperature, then store in an air-tight container.

129 calories per serving
4 gm. fat, 3 gm. protein, 20 gm. carbohydrate,
0 cholesterol, 404 mg. sodium.

For exchange diets, count: 1 1/2 starch.

Fluffy Fruit Dip

Use this dip with apple wedges, pineapple spears,
nectarine slices, or fresh grapes.

Preparation time: 20 minutes
Chilling time: at least 2 hours

8 servings—1/4 cup each

1 cup skim milk
1/2 cup egg substitute or 2 whole eggs
2 tablespoons sugar or 2 tablespoons Nutrasweet
   Spoonfuls
1 teaspoon vanilla
1/8 teaspoon nutmeg
2 tablespoons orange juice
2 teaspoons orange extract
1 cup reduced-fat whipped topping

1. In a small saucepan, use an egg beater to beat together skim milk, egg or egg substitute, and sugar, if you are using it.

2. Heat mixture over medium heat, stirring constantly, about 5 minutes until mixture becomes thick.

3. Remove saucepan from heat, and whisk in Nutrasweet Spoonful (if you're using that instead of sugar), vanilla, and nutmeg. Transfer to a serving bowl, and stir in orange juice and orange extract.

4. Cover and refrigerate for 2 hours. Just before serving, stir in whipped topping.

113 calories per serving (102 calories with sugar substitute)
5 gm. fat, 3 gm. protein (2 gm. protein with sugar substitute),
15 gm. carbohydrate (9 gm. carbohydrate with sugar substitute),
0 cholesterol (54 mg. cholesterol with eggs), 44 mg. sodium.

For exchange diets, count: 1 fruit, 1 fat.

Fruit and Nut Spread for Bagels

Preparation time: 10 minutes

8 servings—1/4 cup each

8 ounces reduced-fat cream cheese, softened
1/2 cup dried fruit bits (recommend dried pineapple,
    apricots, and pears)
1 tablespoon all-fruit spread (any flavor is acceptable)
2 tablespoons chopped pecans

1. Combine all ingredients in a small bowl. Refrigerate in a covered container, and use with cinnamon raisin bagels.

97 calories per serving
4 gm. fat, 4 gm. protein, 14 gm. carbohydrate,
1 mg. cholesterol, 140 mg. sodium.

For exchange diets, count: 1 fruit, 1 fat.

Fred's Pineapple Fruit Dip

Preparation time: 15 minutes
Chilling time: 2 hours

12 servings—1/4 cup each

1 1/2 cups nonfat sour cream
1/3 cup frozen pineapple juice concentrate
1 teaspoon finely grated lime rind
1 cup reduced-fat whipped topping, thawed

1. Combine ingredients in a mixing bowl and stir to mix. Chill at least 2 hours before serving with assorted fresh fruit dippers.

84 calories per serving
3 gm. fat, 2 gm. protein, 13 gm. carbohydrate,
0 cholesterol, 40 mg. sodium.

For exchange diets, count: 1 fruit, 1/2 fat.

Grilled Cheese Sandwich

Preparation time: 15 minutes
Cooking time: 6 minutes

4 servings—1 sandwich each

4 ounces reduced-fat American cheese
8 slices cracked wheat bread
2 teaspoons soft margarine

1. Place the cheese between 2 slices of bread. Spread 1/2 tsp. of margarine on each outside slice.

2. Heat a no-stick skillet over medium heat. Brown the sandwich 2 to 3 minutes on each side, until cheese melts. Add some lettuce, tomato, or cucumber for extra crunch.

240 calories per serving
6 gm. fat, 11 gm. protein, 30 gm. carbohydrate,
0 cholesterol, 710 mg. sodium.

For exchange diets, count: 1 lean meat, 1/2 fat, 2 starch.

Kitchen Quarterback Salsa and Bean Dip

Preparation time: 5 minutes
Cooking time: 6 minutes

8 servings—1/2 cup each

4 ounces reduced-fat processed cheese spread,
   cut into chunks
1/2 cup chunky salsa
16-ounce can fat-free refried beans with green chilies

1. Combine all three ingredients in a microwave safe dish. Cook 6 minutes, stopping to stir the mixture twice during cooking. Serve with reduced-fat tortilla chips.

70 calories per serving
2 gm. fat, 4 gm. protein, 10 gm. carbohydrate,
2 mg. cholesterol, 275 mg. sodium.

For exchange diets, count: 1/2 skim milk, 1 vegetable.

Kids Can Make This Cheesy Bean Dip

Preparation time: 10 minutes
Baking time: 15 minutes

16 servings—1/3 cup each

8 ounces nonfat cream cheese, softened
2 16-ounce cans red beans in hot chili sauce
1/2 cup shredded low-fat cheddar cheese
3 1/2-ounce can diced green chili peppers (drained)

1. Preheat oven to 350°.

2. Spread cream cheese on bottom of 9" x 13" pan. Drain liquid from beans, then spread beans over cream cheese layer. Sprinkle cheddar cheese over beans.

3. Scatter green chilies over cheese.

4. Bake for 15 minutes. Allow to cool slightly before serving (5 to 10 minutes). Serve with reduced-fat crackers or tortilla chips.

90 calories per serving
2 gm. fat, 2 gm. protein, 15 gm. carbohydrate,
8 mg. cholesterol, 458 mg. sodium.

For exchange diets, count: 1 starch

Let Good Times Roll Cheese Ball

Preparation time: 20 minutes
Chilling time: 2 hours

12 servings—3 tablespoons each

8-ounce package reduced-fat cream cheese, softened
1/3 cup crushed pineapple, drained very well
1 green onion, chopped fine
1/4 cup chopped green pepper
1/4 cup chopped pecans
1/2 teaspoon seasoned salt

1. Combine ingredients in a small mixing bowl. Refrigerate at least 2 hours.

49 calories per serving
3 gm. fat, 3 gm. protein, 3 gm. carbohydrate,
0 cholesterol, 56 mg. sodium.

For exchange diets, count: 1/2 fat, 1 vegetable.

Low-Fat Ranch Dip for Veggies

Preparation time: 5 minutes
16 servings—2 tablespoons each

1 cup reduced-fat sour cream
1 cup fat-free mayonnaise or salad dressing
1 envelope buttermilk ranch salad dressing mix

1. Combine ingredients in a small bowl. Cover and refrigerate until use.

35 calories per serving
2 gm. fat, 1 gm. protein, 4 gm. carbohydrate,
5 mg. cholesterol, 330 mg. sodium
(to reduce sodium, use half of salad dressing mix).

For exchange diets, count: 1 vegetable.

Low-Fat Sour Cream 'n Onion Chip Dip

Preparation time: 5 minutes

8 servings—1/4 cup each

1 cup reduced-fat sour cream
1 cup fat-free mayonnaise or salad dressing
1 envelope onion soup mix

serving tip: use baked potato chips as dippers

1. Combine ingredients in a small bowl. Cover and refrigerate until use.

67 calories per serving
0 fat, 3 gm. protein, 14 gm. carbohydrate,
0 cholesterol, 835 mg. sodium
(to reduce sodium, use 1/2 envelope of onion soup mix).

For exchange diets, count: 1/2 skim milk, 1 vegetable.

Low-Fat Cocoa Mix

Preparation time: 15 minutes

22 servings—2 tablespoons of mix each

1/2 cup nonfat coffee creamer
3/4 cup cocoa
1/2 cup nonfat dry milk
sugar substitute equivalent to 1 cup sugar, such as
    Equal Measure

1. Combine all ingredients in a covered container. Mix 2 tablespoons of cocoa mix with 6 ounces boiling water.

22 calories per serving
0 fat, 1 gm. protein, 5 gm. carbohydrate,
0 cholesterol, 13 mg. sodium.

For exchange diets, count: 1/2 fruit.

Marinated Vegetable Appetizers

Preparation time: 15 minutes
Marinating time: 4 hours

12 servings—1/2 cup each

8 ounces fresh mushrooms, cleaned
1 small head broccoli, broken into florets and washed
8 ounces baby carrots, washed
2 tablespoons lemon juice

Marinade:
1 cup fat-free Italian dressing
1 tablespoon grated lemon peel
2 tablespoons sliced pimiento
2 tablespoons chopped fresh parsley

1. Combine vegetables in a microwave-safe shallow dish. Sprinkle with 2 tablespoons of lemon juice. Cover and cook for 3 minutes.

2. Meanwhile, mix ingredients for marinade in a shaker container. Pour marinade over the steamed vegetables. Cover and chill at least 4 hours, stirring vegetables at least twice during the marinating time. Serve vegetables on a platter with toothpicks.

24 calories per serving
0 fat, 1 gm. protein, 6 gm. carbohydrate,
0 cholesterol, 157 mg. sodium.

For exchange diets, count: 1 vegetable.

Onion and Dill Spread for Bagels

Preparation time: 10 minutes

8 servings—1/4 cup each

8 ounces reduced-fat cream cheese, softened
1 tablespoon dill weed
2 green onions, finely chopped
1 tablespoon reduced-sodium soy sauce

1. Combine all ingredients in a small bowl. Refrigerate in a covered container; use with onion bagels. This may be used immediately or stored in the refrigerator for 2 weeks.

22 calories per serving
0 fat, 3 gm. protein, 2 gm. carbohydrate,
1 mg. cholesterol, 212 mg. sodium.

For exchange diets, count: 1 vegetable.

Orange Fruit Sicle

Preparation time: 15 minutes
Freezing time: 2 hours

4 servings—1 sicle each

2 cups nonfat sugar-free vanilla yogurt
6-ounce can frozen orange juice concentrate
1 teaspoon vanilla

1. Combine ingredients in a mixing bowl, then pour into popsicle molds and freeze. Insert sticks when mixture is partially frozen.

86 calories per serving
0 fat, 7 gm. protein, 14 gm. carbohydrate,
3 mg. cholesterol, 88 mg. sodium.

For exchange diets, count: 1/2 fruit, 1/2 skim milk.

Orange Spread for Bagels

Preparation time: 15 minutes

8 servings—1/4 cup each

8 ounces reduced-fat cream cheese, softened
1/2 cup all-fruit orange marmalade

1. Combine cream cheese and marmalade in a small bowl. Refrigerate in a covered container, and use with poppy seed bagels.

65 calories per serving
0 fat, 3 gm. protein, 14 gm. carbohydrate,
1 mg. cholesterol, 93 mg. sodium.

For exchange diets, count: 1 fruit.

Party Hearty Cereal Mix

Preparation time: 15 minutes
Baking time: 1 hour

16 servings—1/2 cup each

1/4 cup soft margarine
1 tablespoon Worcestershire sauce
1 teaspoon hot pepper sauce
1/2 teaspoon seasoned salt
7 cups of your favorite cereal (recommend Crispix or Chex)
1 cup mustard-flavored pretzels

1. Preheat oven to 250°.

2. Combine first four ingredients in a glass measure, and microwave on 50% power for 1 minute or until margarine is melted.

3. Combine cereal and pretzels in a baking pan. Pour margarine and seasonings over the top and stir to mix. Bake for 1 hour, stirring four times during baking. Cool to room temperature, then store in an airtight container.

126 calories per serving
3 gm. fat, 2 gm. protein, 22 gm. carbohydrate,
0 cholesterol, 375 mg. sodium
(to reduce sodium, reduce or omit seasoned salt).

For exchange diets, count: 1 1/2 starch.

Peach Slush

Preparation time: 15 minutes

8 servings—6 ounces each

2 large ripe peaches, with peeling, cut into slices
1 fresh lime, peeled and chopped
1 envelope sugar-free lemon-lime drink powder
3 cups crushed ice
1 tablespoon rum flavoring

1. Combine ingredients in a blender container, process until no chunks of peach or lime remain. Serve immediately.

29 calories per serving
0 fat, 0 protein, 7 gm. carbohydrate,
0 cholesterol, 1 mg. sodium.

For exchange diets, count: 1/2 fruit.

Percolator Fruit Punch

Preparation time: 15 minutes

8 servings—3/4 cup each

2 cups pineapple juice (may substitute orange juice)
2 cups water
2 cups cranberry juice (may substitute cran-raspberry)
1 tablespoon whole cloves
4 cinnamon sticks, broken into pieces
1 1/2 teaspoons whole allspice
1/4 teaspoon salt

1. Combine first three ingredients in a 12-cup percolator. Place spices and salt in the basket. Perk for 10 minutes.

73 calories per serving
0 fat, 0 protein, 18 gm. carbohydrate,
0 cholesterol, 115 mg. sodium.

For exchange diets, count: 1 fruit.

Pink Slush

Preparation time: 10 minutes
Freezing time: 12 hours

16 servings—8 ounce each

12 ounces frozen orange juice concentrate
1 packet sugar-free pink lemonade drink powder
46 ounces pineapple juice
46 ounces apricot nectar
36 ounces (3 12-ounce cans) sugar-free lemon-lime soft
   drink

1. Combine first four ingredients in a large plastic container, and freeze at least 12 hours.

2. One hour before serving, remove from the freezer. Use a heavy, long-handled metal spoon to break up slush for serving. Scoop 6 ounces slush into a short glass and pour in 2 ounces soft drink. Garnish the glass with a melon ball on a swizzle stick.

112 calories per serving
0 fat, 0 protein, 28 gm. carbohydrate,
0 cholesterol, 6 mg. sodium.

For exchange diets, count: 2 fruit.

Salmon Pâté

Preparation time: 15 minutes
Chilling time: at least 6 hours

8 servings—1/4 cup each

16-ounce can pink salmon, well drained and flaked
4 ounces reduced-fat cream cheese, softened
1 green onion, diced fine
1 tablespoon finely grated lemon peel
2 tablespoons fresh lemon juice
1 teaspoon dill weed
1/2 teaspoon seasoned salt
garnish: minced fresh parsley

1. Combine all ingredients in a mixing bowl. Use an electric mixer on low to medium speed to blend, mixing 1 to 2 minutes.

2. Line a 2-cup bowl or mold with plastic wrap. Spoon salmon mixture into the bowl or mold, smoothing the top. Cover and chill 6 hours or overnight. Unmold the pâté onto a serving dish. Remove the plastic wrap and garnish the outside with minced parsley. Serve with reduced-fat crackers.

114 calories per serving
5 gm. fat, 216 gm. protein, 1 gm. carbohydrate,
37 mg. cholesterol, 142 mg. sodium.

For exchange diets, count: 2 lean meat.

Sangria

Preparation time: 10 minutes

8 servings—6 ounces each

juice of 3 fresh oranges
juice of 2 fresh lemons
2 cups grape juice
8 large ice cubes
1 fresh lemon, sliced thin
1 fresh orange, sliced thin
25-ounce bottle sparkling mineral water, chilled

1. Combine orange juice, lemon juice, and grape juice in a large pitcher. Add ice cubes and fruit slices to the pitcher and stir. Slowly pour in sparkling mineral water just before serving.

50 calories per serving
0 fat, 0 protein, 12 gm. carbohydrate,
0 cholesterol, 2 mg. sodium.

For exchange diets, count: 1 fruit.

Shrimp Spread for Bagels

Preparation time: 15 minutes
Chilling time: 2 hours

8 servings—1/4 cup each

8 ounces reduced-fat cream cheese, softened
1/3 cup ketchup
2 tablespoons horseradish
4 ounces cooked shrimp, chopped

1. Combine all ingredients in a small bowl. Refrigerate in a covered container, and use with sesame seed bagels. This spread is best refrigerated for 2 hours before serving and will keep for 3 days.

46 calories per serving
0 fat, 6 gm. protein, 4 gm. carbohydrate,
29 mg. cholesterol, 261 mg. sodium.

For exchange diets, count: 1 vegetable, 1 very lean meat.

Spinach Dip

Preparation time: 15 minutes
Chilling time: 2 hours

12 servings—1/3 cup each

4 strips bacon, diced, cooked crisp, and drained
1 cup plain yogurt
1 1/2 cups reduced-fat mayonnaise or salad dressing
1 teaspoon salt
1 teaspoon dry mustard
2 green onions, chopped
10-ounce package frozen spinach, thawed
   and squeezed dry
8-ounce can sliced water chestnuts

1. Combine all ingredients in a large bowl. Cover and chill for at least 2 hours. Serve with fresh vegetables or chunks of fresh bread.

61 calories per serving
0 fat, 3 gm. protein, 11 gm. carbohydrate,
2 mg. cholesterol, 512 mg. sodium.

For exchange diets, count: 1/2 skim milk, 1 vegetable.

Tortilla Roll-ups

Preparation time: 20 minutes

12 servings—5 rolls each

8 ounces reduced-fat cream cheese, softened
1 cup nonfat sour cream
3 green onions, finely chopped
1 tablespoon dill weed
12 ounces lean ham, diced fine
1 tablespoon dark mustard
12 flour tortillas

1. Combine first six ingredients in a small mixing bowl.

2. Spread cream cheese and ham mixture over the tortillas. Roll up tight, and cut into 5 rolls (about 1 1/2 inch each). Place upright on a serving platter.

136 calories per serving
5 gm. fat, 10 gm. protein, 13 gm. carbohydrate,
16 mg. cholesterol, 639 mg. sodium
(to reduce sodium, use lean turkey instead of ham).

For exchange diets, count: 1 starch, 1 lean meat.

Veggie Pizza Squares

Preparation time: 15 minutes
Baking time: 10 minutes
Cooling time: 20 minutes
Chilling time: 1 hour

24 servings—1/24 of 15" x 8" jelly roll pan

8-roll tube of crescent dinner rolls
Nonstick cooking spray
3 ounces nonfat cream cheese, softened
1/2 cup reduced-fat ranch-type buttermilk
    salad dressing
4 cups assorted raw vegetables, cut in 1/2-inch pieces
(recommend cauliflower, green and red pepper, carrots,
    broccoli)
garnish: chopped fresh chives

1. Preheat oven to 375°.

2. Remove rolls from the tube, and press flat into a 15" x 8" jelly roll pan that has been sprayed with nonstick cooking spray. Pat out to form a crust. Bake for 8 to 10 minutes until lightly browned. Cool crust for 20 minutes.

3. Meanwhile, combine softened cream cheese with salad dressing; and spread over cooled crust. Spread chopped vegetables over dressing and garnish with chives. Refrigerate at least 1 hour or until serving.

52 calories per serving
2 gm. fat, 1 gm. protein, 7 gm. carbohydrate,
1 mg. cholesterol, 166 mg. sodium.

For exchange diets, count: 1 vegetable, 1/2 starch.

Veggie Spread for Bagels

Preparation time: 10 minutes
Chilling time: 2 hours

8 servings—1/4 cup each

8 ounces reduced-fat cream cheese, softened
1/2 carrot, washed and shredded
1 tablespoon dry onion
2 tablespoons minced fresh green pepper
1/2 teaspoon minced garlic
1/2 teaspoon seasoned salt
1/4 cup finely diced fresh cucumber

1. Combine all ingredients in a small bowl. Refrigerate in a covered container, and use with plain bagels. This spread is best chilled for 2 hours and will keep for 1 week.

25 calories per serving
0 fat, 3 gm. protein, 2 gm. carbohydrate,
1 mg. cholesterol, 85 mg. sodium.

For exchange diets, count: 1 vegetable.

Chapter Three

Breads
and
Breakfast

Apple Cinnamon Pull Apart Buns

Preparation time: 20 minutes
Rising time: 1 hour
Baking time: 25 minutes

12 servings—1 bun each

1 pound frozen white bread dough
2 tablespoons reduced-fat margarine
1/2 cup apple juice concentrate
1 teaspoon cinnamon
1/2 cup raisins
1/2 teaspoon cinnamon

1. Defrost bread dough according to package directions.

2. Place margarine in a 9" metal cake pan. Place over low heat until melted. Remove from heat and stir in 1/4 cup of apple juice concentrate and 1 teaspoon cinnamon.

3. Roll dough out on a floured surface into a 12" x 9" rectangle. Drizzle remaining 1/4 cup of apple juice concentrate over the dough. Sprinkle with raisins and 1/2 teaspoon of cinnamon. Roll dough up, jelly-roll fashion, starting with the longest side. Cut crosswise into 12 pieces. Arrange, cut side down, in the prepared pan. Let rise in a warm place for 1 hour or in the refrigerator overnight.

4. Preheat oven to 350°. Bake for 25 minutes until golden brown.

142 calories per serving
2 gm. fat, 4 gm. protein, 26 gm. carbohydrate,
0 cholesterol, 308 mg. sodium.

For exchange diets, count: 1 fruit, 1 starch.

Apple Oat Bran Muffins

Preparation time: 20 minutes
Baking time: 20 minutes

18 servings—1 muffin each

1 1/2 cups flour
1/2 cup Nutrasweet Spoonful sugar substitute
1/2 cup oat bran
1 tablespoon baking power
2 teaspoons cinnamon
1/2 teaspoon salt
1 1/2 cups unsweetened applesauce
1/4 cup skim milk
1/4 cup vegetable oil
1/4 cup frozen apple juice concentrate
1 egg or 1/4 cup liquid egg substitute

Topping:
1 cup dried apple rings, diced fine
1 tablespoon cinnamon

1. Preheat oven to 425°. Fill muffin tins with paper muffin cups.

2. In a mixing bowl, combine flour, sugar substitute, oat bran, baking powder, cinnamon, and salt. Mix well.

3. In another bowl, whisk remaining ingredients together. Pour into the dry ingredients, and stir just until moist. Spoon batter into 18 muffin cups.

4. Mix diced dried apple with cinnamon in a small bowl, and sprinkle on the muffins. Bake for 20 minutes or until muffins test done.

Apple Oat Bran Muffins (continued)

108 calories per serving
4 gm. fat, 3 gm. protein, 19 gm. carbohydrate,
0 cholesterol, 43 mg. sodium.

For exchange diets, count: 1 starch, 1/2 fat.

Banana Nut Crunch Muffins

Preparation time: 20 minutes
Baking time: 20 minutes

12 servings—1 muffin each

nonstick cooking spray
1 1/4 cups bread flour (all-purpose flour is also acceptable)
1 tablespoon baking powder
1/8 teaspoon salt
1 egg or 1/4 cup liquid egg substitute
1/2 cup skim milk
1/4 cup Sugar Twin brown sugar substitute
3 tablespoons vegetable oil
1 1/2 cups Post Banana Nut Crunch cereal
2 large bananas, mashed

Topping:
1/2 cup Post Banana Nut Crunch cereal
1 teaspoon cinnamon

1. Preheat oven to 400°.

2. Prepare muffin pans by lining with paper or spraying with nonstick cooking spray.

3. In a large mixing bowl, combine flour, baking powder, and salt.

4. In a small bowl, combine egg, milk, sugar substitute, and oil. Fold milk mixture into the dry ingredients, and stir, until moist. Fold in cereal and bananas. Spoon into prepared muffin tins.

5. Mix cereal with cinnamon, and sprinkle over the muffins. Bake for 20 minutes or until they are lightly browned.

Banana Nut Crunch Muffins (continued)

104 calories per serving
4 gm. fat, 3 gm. protein, 16 gm. carbohydrate,
0 cholesterol, 27 mg. sodium.

For exchange diets, count: 1 starch, 1/2 fat.

Breakfast for a Bunch

Preparation time: 20 minutes
Baking time: 40 minutes

8 servings—1/8 pan each

nonstick cooking spray
12 slices of white or French bread, crust removed
4 ounces lean cubed ham
2 cups skim milk
8 eggs or 2 cups liquid egg substitute
1/4 cup fresh onion, minced
1/2 teaspoon dry mustard
1/4 teaspoon paprika
1/4 teaspoon salt
1 tablespoon dried parsley

1. Cut bread into cubes and spread over the bottom of a 7" x 11" baking dish that has been sprayed with cooking spray. Sprinkle the ham on the bread.

2. Using a rotary beater, combine the next 6 ingredients in a mixing bowl until well blended. Pour over ham. Sprinkle with parsley. Bake at 400° for 35 to 40 minutes or refrigerate overnight and bake in the morning.

245 calories per serving
7 gm. fat, 17 gm. protein, 22 gm. carbohydrate,
219 mg. cholesterol with eggs (47 mg. with egg substitute),
377 mg. sodium.

For exchange diets, count: 2 lean meat, 1 1/2 starch.

Carrot Bread in the Machine

Preparation time: 10 minutes
Baking time: 4 hours

16 servings—1 slice each

Bread:
    1 cup puréed cooked carrots
    3 tablespoons orange juice
    1 teaspoon margarine
    1 teaspoon salt
    3 cups bread flour
    1 tablespoon sugar
    1 teaspoon cinnamon
    1/4 teaspoon nutmeg
    2 teaspoons bread machine yeast

Add ingredients:
    1/4 cup chopped walnuts

1. Add bread ingredients to the bread machine pan in the order suggested by your manufacturer.

2. Add nuts to the bread during the "Add ingredient" phase, usually about 40 minutes into the cycle.

120 calories per serving
2 gm. fat, 4 gm. protein, 21 gm. carbohydrate,
0 cholesterol, 81 mg. sodium.

For exchange diets, count: 1 1/2 starch.

Cracked Wheat Bread in the Machine

Preparation time: 10 minutes
Baking time: 4 hours

16 servings—1 slice each

1 1/8 cups water
1 teaspoon salt
3 tablespoons nonfat dry milk powder
1 tablespoon sugar
2 cups bread flour
1 cup cracked wheat
2 teaspoons bread machine yeast

1. Add bread ingredients to the bread machine pan in the order suggested by your manufacturer.

111 calories per serving
1 gm. fat, 4 gm. protein, 22 gm. carbohydrate,
3 mg. cholesterol, 79 mg. sodium.

For exchange diets, count: 1 1/2 starch.

Cranberry-Lemon Bread in the Machine

Preparation time: 10 minutes
Baking time: 4 hours

16 servings—1 slice each

3/4 cup skim milk
2 tablespoons freshly squeezed lemon juice
1 whole egg
1 teaspoon margarine
1 teaspoon salt
3 cups bread flour
2 teaspoons sugar
2 teaspoons finely grated lemon peel
2 teaspoons bread machine yeast

Add ingredients:
1/2 cup dried cranberries

1. Add ingredients to the bread machine pan in the order suggested by your manufacturer.

2. Add cranberries during "Add ingredient" phase, usually about 40 minutes into the cycle.

108 calories per serving
0 fat, 4 gm. protein, 20 gm. carbohydrate,
14 mg. cholesterol, 82 mg. sodium.

For exchange diets, count: 1 1/2 starch.

Crunchy Pita Breakfast

Preparation time: 5 minutes

4 servings—1/2 pita each

2 full pita pockets, cut in half
1/4 cup reduced-fat cream cheese
2 cups fresh or dried fruit of choice, chopped
1/4 cup chopped walnuts

1. Stuff pita pockets with cream cheese, fruit, and nuts. Place on a paper napkin, and microwave on high power for 20 seconds.

187 calories per serving
7 gm. fat, 3 gm. protein, 30 gm. carbohydrate,
0 cholesterol, 154 mg. sodium.

For exchange diets, count: 1 starch, 1 fat, 1 fruit.

German Fruit Bread

This sweet tasting yeast bread is full of rum-flavored fruit.

Preparation time: 30 minutes
Standing time: 1 hour
Rising time: 2 hours, 15 minutes
Baking time: 20 minutes

24 servings—1 slice each

1/2 cup diced citron
1/2 cup raisins
1/4 cup diced candied orange peel
1 tablespoon rum extract
1 package active dry yeast
1/4 cup warm water
1/2 cup lukewarm milk, scalded, then cooled
1/4 cup margarine
2 tablespoons sugar
1/2 teaspoon salt
1/4 teaspoon nutmeg
3 eggs or 3/4 cup liquid egg substitute
4 to 4 1/2 cups flour
1/2 cup chopped blanched almonds
1 tablespoon finely grated lemon peel

1. Mix citron, raisins, orange peel, and extract. Let stand at least one hour.

2. Dissolve yeast in warm water in large bowl. Stir in milk, margarine, sugar, salt, nutmeg, eggs, and 2 cups of the flour. Beat until smooth. Stir in brandied fruit mixture, almonds, lemon peel, and enough remaining flour to make dough easy to handle.

3. Turn dough onto lightly floured surface; knead until smooth and elastic, about 5 minutes. Place in greased bowl; turn greased side up. Cover and let rise in warm place until double, about 1 1/2 hours. Punch down dough and divide in half.

4. Press one half into an oval, about 10" x 7". Fold lengthwise in half; press folded edge firmly. Place folded loaf on greased cookie sheet. Repeat with remaining dough. Cover and let rise until double, about 45 minutes. Bake in preheated 375° oven for 20 to 25 minutes until golden brown.

81 calories per serving
2 gm. fat, 3 gm. protein, 18 gm. carbohydrate,
22 mg. cholesterol with eggs (0 with egg substitute),
136 mg. sodium.

For exchange diets, count: 1 starch.

Golden Morning Muffins

Preparation time: 20 minutes
Baking time: 25 minutes

24 servings—1 muffin each

2 cups flour
1 cup cornmeal
5 teaspoons baking powder
1 teaspoon salt
1/2 cup sugar
1/2 cup vegetable oil
2 eggs or 1/2 cup liquid egg substitute
1/2 cup orange juice concentrate
1 cup skim milk
7-ounce can crushed pineapple, drained well
1/2 cup freshly grated carrots

1. Preheat oven to 425°.

2. In a mixing bowl, combine first four ingredients, and mix well.

3. In another mixing bowl, beat sugar, oil, eggs, orange juice concentrate, and milk until smooth. Make a well in the dry ingredients, and pour in egg and oil mixture. Stir just until moist. Gently fold in drained pineapple and grated carrots.

4. Line muffin tins with paper liners. Divide muffin batter between 24 cups. Bake for 20 to 25 minutes.

144 calories per serving
5 gm. fat, 3 gm. protein, 23 gm. carbohydrate,
18 mg. cholesterol with eggs (1 mg. cholesterol with egg substitute),
110 mg. sodium.

For exchange diets, count: 1 starch, 1 fruit.

Green Chili Bread with Salsa Spread

Preparation time: 20 minutes
Baking time: 16 minutes

12 servings—1 wedge each

nonstick cooking spray
1 cup quick oats
1 1/4 cups flour
2 teaspoons baking powder
1 teaspoon soda
1/2 teaspoon ground cumin
1/2 teaspoon chili powder
1/2 teaspoon salt
2 tablespoons margarine
2 green onions, diced fine
1/4 cup chopped green chilies
1 cup nonfat sour cream
1 egg

Salsa spread:
    4 ounces nonfat cream cheese, softened
    2 tablespoons mild salsa

1. Preheat oven to 425°.

2. Spray a 10" round cake pan with nonstick cooking spray.

3. In a large bowl, combine dry ingredients, mixing well. Cut in margarine with a pastry blender until mixture resembles coarse crumbs. Stir in onion, sour cream, and egg, mixing just until dry ingredients are moist. Pat dough gently into prepared pan, and bake for 16 minutes until top is golden brown.

Green Chili Bread with Salsa Spread (continued)

4. To prepare spread, combine softened cream cheese with salsa in a small bowl. Cut bread into wedges and serve with salsa spread.

106 calories per serving
2 gm. fat, 5 gm. protein, 18 gm. carbohydrate,
8 mg. cholesterol, 278 mg. sodium.

For exchange diets, count: 1/2 fat, 1 starch.

Hawaii Bread in the Machine

Preparation time: 10 minutes
Baking time: 4 hours

16 servings—1 slice each

Bread:
    3/4 cup milk
    1/4 cup frozen pineapple juice concentrate
    1 egg
    1 teaspoon margarine
    1/2 teaspoon salt
    3 cups flour
    1 tablespoon sugar
    2 teaspoons bread machine yeast

Add ingredients:
    1/4 cup chopped macadamia nuts
    1/4 cup dried coconut

1. Add bread ingredients to the bread machine pan in the order suggested by your manufacturer.

2. Add nuts and coconut to the bread during the "Add ingredient" phase, usually about 40 minutes into the cycle.

149 calories per serving
5 gm. fat, 4 gm. protein, 22 gm. carbohydrate,
14 mg. cholesterol, 49 mg. sodium.

For exchange diets, count: 1 starch, 1 fruit.

Low-Fat French Toast

Preparation time: 10 minutes
Baking time: 20 minutes

4 servings—2 slices each

2 eggs or 1/2 cup liquid egg substitute
1/2 cup skim milk
1/2 teaspoon vanilla
1 teaspoon oil
8 slices bread (best French toast will be from
   sourdough bread that has been allowed to dry out)

1. In a shallow bowl, mix eggs, milk, and vanilla with a fork until smooth.

2. Pour oil into a nonstick skillet and heat over medium-high heat. Use a pastry brush if necessary to coat surface of pan with oil. Reduce heat to medium.

3. Dip the bread into the egg mixture, and place in skillet. Brown both sides of bread, and top with your choice of sugar-free fruit preserves.

193 calories per serving
5 gm. fat, 4 gm. protein, 30 gm. carbohydrate,
137 mg. cholesterol with eggs (0 with egg substitute),
358 mg. sodium.

For exchange diets, count: 2 starch, 1 fat.

Low-Fat Pancakes

Preparation time: 10 minutes
Baking time: 20 minutes

4 servings—2 pancakes each

1 1/2 cups reduced-fat baking mix
1 egg or 1/4 cup liquid egg substitute
1/2 cup skim milk
1/2 teaspoon vanilla
1 teaspoon oil

1. In a mixing bowl, mix baking mix with egg , milk, and vanilla until smooth.

2. Pour oil into a nonstick skillet, and heat over medium-high heat. Use a pastry brush if necessary to coat surface of pan with oil. Reduce heat to medium.

3. Pour 1/4 cup of batter into skillet, and cook until bubbles form. Turn pancake and brown on other side. Top with your choice of sugar-free fruit preserves.

137 calories per serving
6 gm. fat, 3 gm. protein, 15 gm. carbohydrate,
69 mg. cholesterol with eggs (0 with egg substitute),
220 mg. sodium.

For exchange diets, count: 1 starch, 1 fat.

Maple Date Pecan Bread in the Machine

Preparation time: 10 minutes
Baking time: 4 hours

16 servings—1 slice each

Bread:
    1 cup water
    2 tablespoons sugar-free maple syrup
    1 teaspoon maple flavoring
    1 teaspoon margarine
    1 teaspoon salt
    3 tablespoons nonfat dry milk
    3 cups bread flour
    2 teaspoons bread machine yeast

Add ingredients:
    1/3 cup chopped dates
    1/4 cup chopped pecans

1. Add bread ingredients to the bread machine pan in the order suggested by your manufacturer.

2. Add dates and pecans to the bread during the "Add ingredient" phase, usually about 40 minutes into the cycle.

141 calories per serving
3 gm. fat, 4 gm. protein, 25 gm. carbohydrate,
0 cholesterol, 77 mg. sodium.

For exchange diets, count: 1 starch, 1 fruit.

Mashed Potato Bread with Chives in the Machine

Preparation time: 10 minutes
Baking time: 4 hours

16 servings—1 slice each

Bread:
    1 cup mashed potatoes
    1/4 cup milk
    1 teaspoon margarine
    1 teaspoon salt
    3 cups bread flour
    1 teaspoon sugar
    2 teaspoons bread machine yeast

Add ingredients:
    2 tablespoons diced fresh chives

1. Add bread ingredients to the bread machine pan in the order suggested by your manufacturer.

2. Add chives to the bread during the "Add ingredient" phase, usually about 40 minutes into the cycle.

106 calories per serving
1 gm. fat, 3 gm. protein, 21 gm. carbohydrate,
2 mg. cholesterol, 110 mg. sodium.

For exchange diets, count: 1 1/2 starch.

Onion and Poppy Seed Bread in the Machine

Preparation time: 10 minutes
Baking time: 4 hours

16 servings—1 slice each

Bread:
>   3/4 cup nonfat sour cream
>   1/4 cup water
>   1 whole egg
>   1 teaspoon margarine
>   1 teaspoon salt
>   3 cups bread flour
>   2 teaspoons sugar
>   2 teaspoons poppy seed
>   2 teaspoons bread machine yeast

Add ingredients:
>   1/4 cup dried onion
>   2 teaspoons soft margarine

1. Add bread ingredients to the bread machine pan in the order suggested by your manufacturer.

2. Combine dried onion with margarine in a skillet over medium heat; brown onion for 10 to 15 minutes. Add onion to the bread during the "Add ingredient" phase, usually about 40 minutes into the cycle.

119 calories per serving
1 gm. fat, 5 gm. protein, 23 gm. carbohydrate,
13 mg. cholesterol, 96 mg. sodium.

For exchange diets, count: 1 1/2 starch.

Pear and Lemon Bread in the Machine

Preparation time: 10 minutes
Baking time: 4 hours

16 servings—1 slice each

Bread:
   1 cup puréed fresh or juice-packed pears
   2 tablespoons lemon juice
   1 teaspoon margarine
   1 teaspoon salt
   3 cups bread flour
   1 tablespoon brown sugar
   1/2 teaspoon nutmeg
   2 teaspoons finely grated lemon peel
   2 teaspoons bread machine yeast

1. Add bread ingredients to the bread machine pan in the order suggested by your manufacturer.

108 calories per serving
0 fat, 3 gm. protein, 22 gm. carbohydrate,
0 cholesterol, 72 mg. sodium.

For exchange diets, count: 1 1/2 starch.

Pineapple Orange Bread in the Machine

Preparation time: 10 minutes
Baking time: 4 hours

16 servings—1 slice each

Bread:
  3/4 cup milk
  1/4 cup orange juice concentrate
  1 egg
  1 teaspoon margarine
  1/2 teaspoon salt
  3 1/4 cups flour
  1/3 cup cornmeal
  1 tablespoon sugar
  2 teaspoons finely grated orange peel
  2 teaspoons bread machine yeast

Add ingredients:
  1/3 cup diced dried pineapple

1. Add bread ingredients to the bread machine pan in the order suggested by your manufacturer.

2. Add pineapple to the bread during the "Add ingredient" phase, usually about 40 minutes into the cycle.

127 calories per serving
0 fat, 4 gm. protein, 25 gm. carbohydrate,
14 mg. cholesterol, 48 mg. sodium.

For exchange diets, count: 1 1/2 starch.

Pineapple Bran Muffins

Preparation time: 20 minutes
Baking time: 20 minutes

12 servings—1 muffin each

1 cup bran cereal, divided
1 cup dried pineapple, cut into bite-size pieces
1 cup boiling apple juice
3 tablespoons vegetable oil
1 teaspoon vanilla
1 cup flour
1/4 cup sugar or 1/4 cup Sugar Twin
1/2 teaspoon baking soda

1. Preheat oven to 375°.

2. In a large bowl, combine 1/2 cup bran cereal, pineapple bits, and boiling apple juice. Stir in vegetable oil and vanilla.

3. In a small mixing bowl, combine remaining 1/2 cup bran cereal, flour sugar or sugar substitute, and baking soda. Stir in fruit mixture just until moist. Spoon into prepared muffin cups and bake for 25 minutes. Cool on a wire rack.

184 calories per serving (158 calories with sugar substitute)
4 gm. fat, 2 gm. protein, 35 gm. carbohydrate (30 gm. carbohydrate with sugar substitute), 0 cholesterol, 110 mg. sodium.

For exchange diets, count: 2 starch, 1/2 fat.
(Count 2 starch with sugar substitute.)

Poppy Seed Surprise

Preparation time: 20 minutes
Baking time: 55 minutes

36 servings—1 slice each

nonstick cooking spray
3 cups flour
1/2 teaspoon salt
1 1/2 teaspoons baking powder
2/3 cup sugar
2 teaspoons vanilla
1 1/2 cups skim milk
3/4 cup vegetable oil
1/2 cup frozen orange juice concentrate, thawed
2 tablespoons poppy seeds
3 eggs or 3/4 cup liquid egg substitute
1 1/2 teaspoons almond extract
1/2 cup all-fruit raspberry preserves
1 tablespoon finely grated orange rind

1. Preheat oven to 350°. Spray 2 loaf pans with cooking spray.

2. Put all ingredients except raspberry preserves and orange rind into a bowl. Beat for 2 minutes. Spread half of batter over the bottom of the loaf pans.

3. In a small bowl, combine preserves with orange rind. Drizzle preserves over the layer of batter. Spread remaining batter over the preserves. Bake for 55 minutes. Remove from pan and cool on a wire rack.

115 calories per serving
5 gm. fat, 2 gm. protein, 15 gm. carbohydrate,
18 mg. cholesterol (0 cholesterol with egg substitute), 45 mg. sodium.

For exchange diets, count: 1 starch, 1 fat.

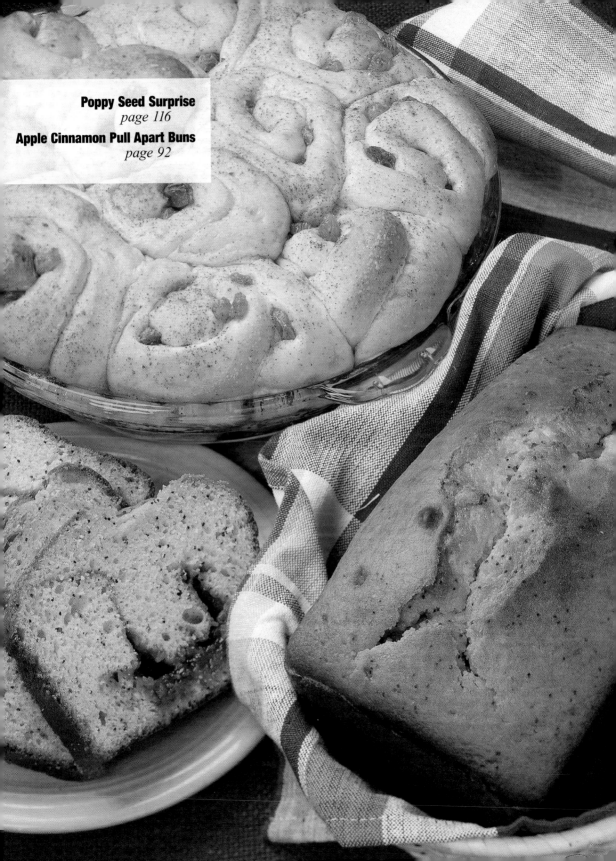

Poppy Seed Surprise
page 116

Apple Cinnamon Pull Apart Buns
page 92

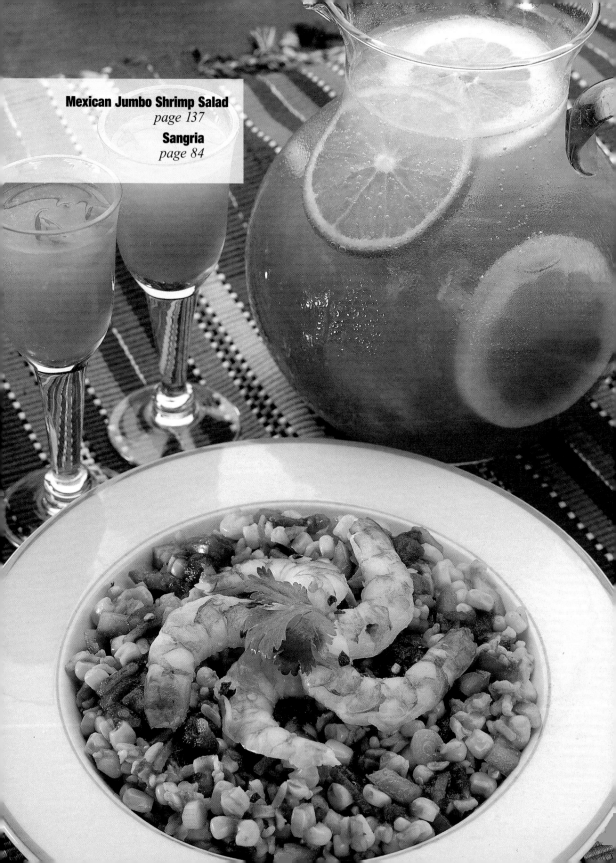

Mexican Jumbo Shrimp Salad
page 137

Sangria
page 84

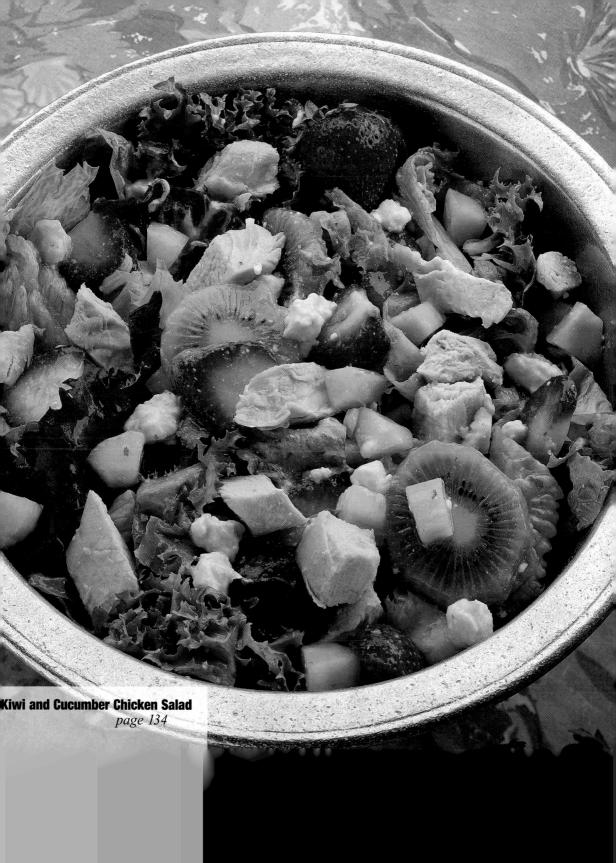

Kiwi and Cucumber Chicken Salad
page 134

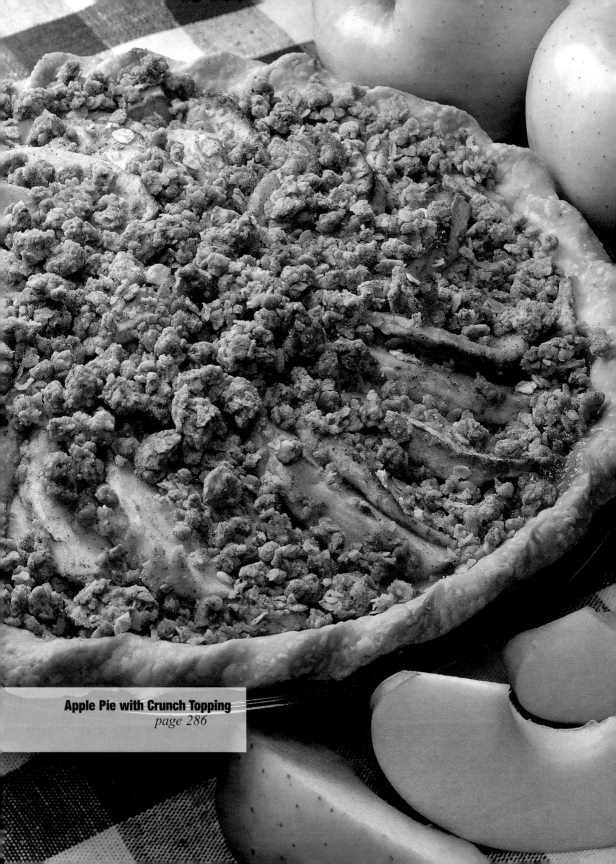

Apple Pie with Crunch Topping
page 286

Pumpkin Nut Bread in the Machine

Preparation time: 10 minutes
Baking time: 4 hours

16 servings—1 slice each

Bread:
  3/4 cup canned pumpkin
  1/3 cup skim milk
  1 egg
  1 teaspoon margarine
  1 teaspoon salt
  3 tablespoons nonfat dry milk
  2 tablespoons brown sugar
  2 teaspoons pumpkin pie spice
  2 1/2 cups bread flour
  2 teaspoons bread machine yeast

Add ingredients:
  1/4 cup chopped pecans

1. Add bread ingredients to the bread machine pan in the order suggested by your manufacturer.

2. Add pecans to the bread during the "Add ingredient" phase, usually about 40 minutes into the cycle.

123 calories per serving
3 gm. fat, 4 gm. protein, 20 gm. carbohydrate,
14 mg. cholesterol, 84 mg. sodium.

For exchange diets, count: 1 1/2 starch.

Scrambled Eggs and Cheese

Preparation time: 15 minutes

4 servings—1/3 cup each

4 eggs or 1 cup liquid egg substitute
1/4 cup skim milk
1/4 teaspoon dried basil
nonstick cooking spray
4 ounces part-skim mozzarella cheese, shredded

1. Combine eggs and milk in a small mixing bowl. Beat well and add dried basil.

2. Spray a no-stick skillet with cooking spray, and heat over medium heat. Pour in egg mixture, and use a spatula to bring cooked portion up from bottom of pan. Sprinkle cheese over eggs just as they become completely firm. Serve as soon as cheese melts.

140 calories per serving
8 gm. fat, 12 gm. protein, 4 gm. carbohydrate,
199 mg. cholesterol (27 mg. cholesterol with egg substitute),
175 mg. sodium.

For exchange diets, count: 1 lean meat, 1/2 skim milk, 1 fat.

Skinny Quiche Lorraine

Preparation time: 10 minutes
Baking time: 30 minutes

8 servings—1 slice each

4 slices bacon, diced
nonstick cooking spray
4 ounces reduced-fat Swiss cheese, shredded
3 green onions, chopped
4-ounce can mushroom pieces, drained
   or 1/2 cup sliced fresh mushrooms
2 1/4 cups skim milk
1 cup reduced-fat baking mix
2 eggs, beaten well, or 1/2 cup liquid egg substitute
1/4 teaspoon pepper

1. Preheat oven to 400°.

2. Dice bacon onto a microwave tray. Cover with a paper towel and cook on high power for 3 minutes. Drain.

3. Spray a 9" pie plate with cooking spray. Sprinkle bacon pieces, shredded cheese, onion, and mushrooms over the pie plate.

4. Beat the remaining ingredients until smooth in the blender or with the electric mixer. Pour into pie. Bake for 30 minutes or until eggs are set.

135 calories per serving
5 gm. fat, 3 gm. protein, 15 gm. carbohydrate,
80 mg. cholesterol (11 mg. cholesterol with egg substitute),
406 mg. sodium.

For exchange diets, count: 1 starch, 1 fat.

Chapter Four

Soups
and
Main-Dish
Salads

Aromatic Chili

Preparation time: 15 minutes
Cooking time: 35 minutes

8 servings—1 1/2 cups each

1 pound lean ground beef, pork, or turkey
1 teaspoon black pepper
1 large red onion, chopped
28-ounce can stewed tomatoes
1 large green pepper, chopped
8 ounces fresh mushrooms, sliced
4 stalks celery, chopped
1 small can diced green chilies
8-ounce can tomato sauce
2 teaspoons chili powder
1 teaspoon allspice
1/4 teaspoon cinnamon
1/2 teaspoon garlic powder
16-ounce can hot chili beans

1. Brown ground meat in a large stockpot. Add black pepper. Pour off any excess fat when done. Add remaining ingredients and bring to a boil. Reduce heat to a simmer, and continue cooking for 25 minutes.

180 calories per serving
2 gm. fat, 18 gm. protein, 24 gm. carbohydrate,
37 mg. cholesterol, 710 mg. sodium
(*to reduce sodium, use no-added-salt tomatoes and tomato sauce*).

For exchange diets, count: 2 very lean meat,
1 starch, 1 vegetable.

Black Bean Soup

Preparation time: 10 minutes
Cooking time: 2 1/2 hours

8 servings—1 cup each

1 pound dry black beans
3 quarts water
4 ounces lean roast beef, shredded
1 large carrot, scrubbed and sliced
1 large white onion, chopped fine
4 whole cloves
1/8 teaspoon red pepper

1/2 cup sherry
1 tablespoon lemon juice
garnish: chopped hard-boiled egg whites

1. Place first seven ingredients in a large stockpot. Bring mixture to a boil. Cover and cook slowly for 2 1/2 hours or until beans are very soft.

2. Remove half of the mixture to a blender container, and process until almost smooth. Return the puréed portion to the stockpot. Stir in sherry and lemon juice, and serve. Garnish with chopped hard-boiled egg whites if desired.

113 calories per serving
1 gm. fat, 8 gm. protein, 13 gm. carbohydrate,
11 mg. cholesterol, 295 mg. sodium.

For exchange diets, count: 1 starch, 1 very lean meat.

Cheesy Fresh Vegetable Soup

Preparation time: 15 minutes
Chilling time: 20 minutes

8 servings—1 cup each

4 cups diced raw vegetables (suggest combination of potatoes, carrots, celery, onion, broccoli, brussel sprouts, cauliflower, asparagus)
1 chicken bouillon cube
1 cup water
13-ounce can reduced-fat cream of chicken soup
1 1/2 cups skim milk
4 ounces reduced-fat American processed cheese, cubed
Garnish: crunchy breadsticks

1. Combine vegetables, water, and bouillon cube in a stockpot. Bring to a boil, then reduce heat; simmer for 20 minutes. Add chicken soup and milk. Bring to a boil, then stir in cheese. Serve when cheese is melted. Garnish with crunchy breadsticks.

122 calories per serving
4 gm. fat, 8 gm. protein, 17 gm. carbohydrate,
4 mg. cholesterol, 769 mg. sodium
(*to reduce sodium, choose no-added-salt bouillon*).

For exchange diets, count: 1 starch, 2 vegetable.

Clam Chowder

Preparation time: 15 minutes
Cooking time: 40 minutes

8 servings—1 cup each

4 strips bacon
2 ribs celery, diced fine
1 small onion, diced
2 (8-ounce) cans minced clams with juice
2 cups evaporated skim milk
2 large potatoes, peeled and diced
1/2 teaspoon pepper
1 teaspoon butter-flavored sprinkles,
    such as Molly McButter

1. In a Dutch oven, cook bacon with celery and onion until bacon is crisp. Spoon drippings from the pan, then drain the bacon and vegetables between two paper towels. Return the bacon and the vegetables to the pot.

2. Add all remaining ingredients and cook over medium-low heat for 30 minutes or until the potatoes are tender. Do not boil this soup vigorously, as the creamy texture will be lost.

117 calories per serving
1 gm. fat, 6 gm. protein, 20 gm. carbohydrate,
4 mg. cholesterol, 342 mg. sodium.

For exchange diets, count: 1 starch, 1/2 skim milk.

Cream Soup Substitute

Preparation time: 10 minutes

10 batches—equivalent to 1 (15-ounce) can cream soup each

2 cups nonfat dried milk
3/4 cup cornstarch
1/4 cup chicken or beef bouillon particles
2 tablespoons dried minced onion
1 teaspoon thyme
1 teaspoon basil
1/2 teaspoon pepper

1. Mix ingredients together and store in a covered container. Use as a substitute for creamed soups in casserole recipes.

2. To use, mix 1 1/4 cups cold water with 1/3 cup of the mix in a small saucepan. Add 1 teaspoon margarine. Cook until thickened. Substitute for a 15-ounce can of cream soup.

94 calories per batch
0 fat, 2 gm. protein, 14 gm. carbohydrate,
3 mg. cholesterol, 112 mg. sodium.

For exchange diets, count: 1 starch.

Deli Salad

Preparation time: 20 minutes
Marinating time: 30 minutes recommended

8 servings—1 1/2 cup each

8 ounces rotini
8-ounce can artichoke hearts, drained and chopped
4 ounces Canadian bacon, sliced
3 cups your favorite chopped vegetables (use cauliflower, broccoli,
   carrots, peppers, onions, mushrooms, zucchini, summer squash, or
   whatever you have on hand)
2 green onions, diced fine
1 cup fat-free Italian dressing
1 ounce freshly grated Parmesan cheese

1. Prepare rotini according to package directions, and drain well.

2. Combine drained rotini with all remaining ingredients in a large salad
bowl; toss to mix. Serve immediately or improve the flavor by marinating in
the refrigerator for at least 30 minutes.

164 calories per serving
3 gm. fat, 10 gm. protein, 27 gm. carbohydrate,
9 mg. cholesterol, 709 mg. sodium
(to reduce sodium, use turkey instead of Canadian bacon).

For exchange diets, count: 1 starch, 1 lean meat, 1 vegetable.

Fish and Mixed Vegetable Stew

Crab is the richest seafood source of zinc—5 mg. per 3-ounce portion.

Preparation time: 15 minutes
Cooking time: 20 minutes

8 servings—1 cup each

1 medium onion, chopped
1 teaspoon vegetable oil
28-ounce can whole tomatoes
2 medium potatoes, peeled and diced
1/2 teaspoon basil
1/4 teaspoon pepper
1/2 teaspoon sugar
1 1/2 pound fresh or frozen crab meat,
    flaked into bite-size pieces
16 ounces frozen mixed vegetables

1. Sauté onion in oil until tender in a 4-quart saucepan. Stir in tomatoes. Add potatoes, basil, pepper, and sugar, and cook over high heat until boiling. Reduce heat to low, cover and simmer for another 15 minutes or until potatoes are tender. Stir occasionally.

2. Meanwhile, flake crab into bite-size pieces. Add crab and frozen vegetables to tomato mixture, and heat just until boiling. Reduce heat to low, cover, and simmer for 8 minutes or until vegetables and crab are tender when tested with a fork.

165 calories per serving
2 gm. fat, 19 gm. protein, 20 gm. carbohydrate,
35 mg. cholesterol, 893 mg. sodium
(to reduce sodium, use no-added-salt tomatoes
and reduced-sodium crab).

For exchange diets, count: 2 very lean meat,
1 starch, 1 vegetable.

Gazpacho

Preparation time: 15 minutes
Chilling time: 30 minutes

8 servings—3/4 cup each

3 cloves fresh garlic, minced
3 tablespoons white vinegar
1/2 teaspoon salt
1 teaspoon vegetable oil
1 teaspoon tarragon
1 teaspoon Nutrasweet Spoonful sugar substitute
24-ounce can vegetable juice cocktail, divided
1 large green pepper, halved and seeded
1 large cucumber, pared
2 ribs of celery
2 medium tomatoes, peeled and quartered

1. Combine minced garlic, vinegar, salt, oil, tarragon, sugar substitute, and 2 cups of vegetable juice cocktail in a large bowl.

2. In a blender or food processor, process pepper, cucumber, celery, tomatoes, and 1 cup of the vegetable juice cocktail until finely chopped. Add to garlic and vinegar mixture. Chill at least 30 minutes. Ladle into bowls, and serve with breadsticks.

44 calories per serving
0 fat, 1 gm. protein, 9 gm. carbohydrate,
0 cholesterol, 424 mg. sodium.

For exchange diets, count: 2 vegetable.

Ham and Cheddar Soup

Kids will love this as much as a ham and cheese sandwich.

Preparation time: 15 minutes
Cooking time: 20 minutes

8 servings—1 cup each

2 cups no-added-salt chicken broth
2 large potatoes, peeled and diced
1 large carrot, peeled and cut into coins
1 rib celery, cleaned and diced
1 small onion, chopped
1/2 teaspoon salt
1/2 teaspoon white pepper

Thickening:
    1/4 cup flour
    2 cups skim milk
    4 ounces reduced-fat cheddar cheese, shredded
    4 ounces very lean ham, cubed

1. Combine broth, vegetables, salt, and pepper in a stockpot. Bring to a boil, then reduce heat and simmer for 10 minutes.

2. Meanwhile, combine flour and milk in a shaker container. Slowly pour thickening into the vegetable mixture. Use a whisk to blend well. Bring mixture back to a boil, then reduce heat to low and stir in cheese and ham. Serve when cheese is melted.

79 calories per serving
0 fat, 4 gm. protein, 15 gm. carbohydrate,
1 mg. cholesterol, 126 mg. sodium.

For exchange diets, count: 1 starch.

Ham and Cheese Chef Salad

Preparation time: 20 minutes

4 servings—3 cups each

4 ounces lean ham, cut into thin strips
2 medium heads Boston lettuce, torn into bite-size pieces
2 ounces reduced-fat Swiss cheese, shredded
1/2 cup dried cherries or 1/2 cup diced dried apple rings

Dressing:
1 tablespoon olive oil
1/4 cup red wine vinegar
2 tablespoons apple juice
1/2 teaspoon minced garlic
1/2 teaspoon black pepper

1. Combine ham, lettuce, Swiss cheese, and fruit in a large salad bowl.

2. Combine ingredients for the dressing in a shaker container, and shake
to mix. Pour dressing over the salad and toss. Serve on chilled salad
plates with hot breadsticks.

148 calories per serving
9 gm. fat, 10 gm. protein, 7 gm. carbohydrate,
28 mg. cholesterol, 353 mg. sodium.

For exchange diets, count: 1 fat, 1 lean meat, 2 vegetable.

Hamburger Veggie Soup

Preparation time: 20 minutes
Cooking time: 30 minutes

8 servings—1 1/2 cups each

1 pound lean ground beef
1 large white onion, peeled and diced
1 large potato, peeled and diced
1 cup shredded cabbage
2 (14-ounce) cans chunky tomatoes
16-ounce can no-added-salt beef broth
1/2 teaspoon thyme
1/2 teaspoon basil
1/2 teaspoon salt
1/2 teaspoon pepper
1 tablespoon Worcestershire sauce
1 bay leaf

1. In a large Dutch oven, brown ground beef with onions over medium heat until meat is no longer pink. Drain meat well, and return it to the Dutch oven.

2. Add all remaining ingredients. Bring the mixture to a boil, then reduce heat to simmer for 15 minutes or until the vegetables are tender.

196 calories per serving
8 gm. fat, 20 gm. protein, 12 gm. carbohydrate,
57 mg. cholesterol, 702 mg. sodium
(to reduce sodium, omit salt and use no-added-salt tomatoes).

For exchange diets, count: 1 vegetable, 1/2 starch, 3 lean meat.

Italian Beef and Vegetable Soup

Preparation time: 20 minutes
Cooking time: 25 minutes

8 servings—1 1/4 cups each

1/2 pound lean ground beef
1/2 teaspoon minced garlic
1/2 teaspoon pepper
1/4 teaspoon salt
2 (14-ounce) cans no-added-salt beef broth
14-ounce can Italian-style seasoned tomatoes
16-ounce can cannellini (white kidney) beans, rinsed and drained
1 large carrot, washed and cut into coins
2 small zucchini, washed and cut into coins

1. In a Dutch oven, brown ground beef with garlic, pepper, and salt over medium heat until meat is no longer pink. Drain well.

2. Add all remaining ingredients. Bring mixture to a boil, then reduce heat and simmer for 10 minutes.

148 calories per serving
5 gm. fat, 12 gm. protein, 13 gm. carbohydrate,
24 mg. cholesterol, 920 mg. sodium
(to reduce sodium, omit salt and use no-added-salt
Italian-style tomatoes).

For exchange diets, count: 1 lean meat, 1 starch.

Kiwi and Cucumber Chicken Salad

Preparation time: 20 minutes

4 servings—2 cups each

4 cups mixed salad greens
3 kiwifruit, peeled and sliced
2 skinless, boneless chicken breasts, cooked and diced
1 small cucumber, peeled, seeded, and diced
1 cup sliced strawberries
1/4 cup crumbled feta cheese
1/2 cup reduced-fat vinaigrette salad dressing

1. Combine all ingredients in a large salad bowl. Toss and serve.

215 calories per serving
6 gm. fat, 20 gm. protein, 23 gm. carbohydrate,
49 mg. cholesterol, 211 mg. sodium.

For exchange diets, count: 2 lean meat, 1 fruit, 2 vegetable.

Lemon Chicken Salad

Preparation time: 20 minutes
Chilling time: 1 hour

8 servings—1/4 cup each

1/4 cup reduced-fat mayonnaise
1/4 cup nonfat sour cream
1 teaspoon fresh grated lemon peel
1 teaspoon lemon juice
1/2 teaspoon salt
1/4 teaspoon white pepper
4 (3-ounce) chicken breasts, cooked through and diced
  (approximately 3 cups of meat)
2 large ribs celery, diced fine
2 green onions, diced fine

1. In a large salad bowl, combine all ingredients in order listed. Cover and chill for at least 1 hour or until serving time. This salad is good accompanied by reduced-fat crackers and fresh fruit.

160 calories per serving
6 gm. fat, 30 gm. protein, 4 gm. carbohydrate,
86 mg. cholesterol, 465 mg. sodium.

For exchange diets, count: 4 lean meat, 1 vegetable.

Long-Cook Ham and Bean Soup

Preparation time: 15 minutes
Cooking time: 2 1/2 hours

8 servings—1 cup each

2 cups dry navy or pinto beans
2 quarts water
4 ounces lean ham, shredded
1 small onion, diced
1 teaspoon salt
1 bay leaf
3 tablespoons Worcestershire sauce
3 large carrots, scrubbed and sliced thin

1. In a large stockpot, combine all ingredients except the carrots, and bring to a boil. Reduce heat to simmer. Cover, and cook for 2 1/2 hours or until beans are tender.

2. Add the carrots 30 minutes before the end of the cooking time to ensure a favorable texture.

215 calories per serving
2 gm. fat, 15 gm. protein, 35 gm. carbohydrate,
8 mg. cholesterol, 510 mg. sodium
(to reduce sodium, omit salt).

For exchange diets, count: 1 very lean meat,
1 vegetable, 1 1/2 starch.

Mexican Jumbo Shrimp Salad

Preparation time: 20 minutes

4 servings—1 1/2 cups each

1 cup instant brown rice
3/4 cup no-added-salt chicken broth
14-ounce can whole kernel corn, drained well
1 green pepper, diced
1 green onion, finely chopped
1/2 cup mild salsa
1 tablespoon lime juice
1/2 teaspoon finely grated lime peel
1/2 teaspoon cumin
8 ounces jumbo shrimp, peeled, cooked chilled, and
    halved lengthwise
red pepper

1. In a microwave-safe dish, combine instant brown rice and chicken broth. Cover and cook for 4 minutes. Remove cover, and stir in 2 large ice cubes to speed cooling.

2. Meanwhile, combine corn, peppers, green onion, and salsa in a salad bowl.

3. In a shaker container, mix salsa, lime juice, lime peel, and cumin. Add the cooled rice to the corn, then pour salsa mixture on top. Toss to mix.

4. Divide rice mixture among 4 salad plates, and arrange shrimp on top. Garnish with a dash of red pepper.

255 calories per serving
3 gm. fat, 19 gm. protein, 43 gm. carbohydrate,
87 mg. cholesterol, 546 mg. sodium.
(to reduce sodium, use no-added-salt corn and salsa).

For exchange diets, count: 2 starch,
1 vegetable, 2 very lean meat.

Minestrone

Preparation time: 15 minutes
Cooking time: 25 minutes

8 servings—1 1/2 cups each

1 tablespoon olive oil
1/4 teaspoon minced garlic
1 large onion, chopped fine
2 ribs celery with leaves, chopped fine
1 large carrot, washed and sliced thin
16-ounce-can chunky tomatoes with Italian seasoning
16-ounce-can red kidney beans, drained and rinsed
1 quart no-added-salt beef broth
6-ounce-can tomato paste
1 ounce spaghetti noodles, broken into small pieces

1. In a large Dutch oven, sauté garlic, onion, and celery in olive oil over medium heat until vegetables are tender. Add all remaining ingredients except the spaghetti. Bring mixture to a boil, then reduce heat to a simmer for at least 15 minutes or up to 1 hour. Add spaghetti during last 8 minutes of simmering.

119 calories per serving
2 gm. fat, 6 gm. protein, 20 gm. carbohydrate,
0 cholesterol, 976 mg. sodium
(to reduce sodium, use no-added-salt tomatoes and tomato paste).

For exchange diets, count: 1 starch, 2 vegetable.

Mulligatawny Soup

Curry is an ancient treatment for respiratory disease.

Preparation time: 15 minutes
Cooking time: 25 minutes

8 servings—1 cup each

1/4 cup chopped onion
1/2 teaspoon curry powder
1 tablespoon margarine
1 cup cooked, diced chicken
1 small tart apple, peeled, cored, and chopped
1/2 cup shredded carrot
1/4 cup chopped celery
2 tablespoons chopped green pepper
3 tablespoons flour
4 cups no-added-salt chicken broth
16-ounce can no-added-salt chunky tomatoes
2 teaspoons lemon juice
1 1/2 teaspoons dried parsley
   or 1 1/2 tablespoons minced fresh parsley
1 teaspoon sugar
2 whole cloves

1. In a large stockpot, cook onion and curry powder in margarine until onion is tender. Stir in chicken, chopped apple, carrot, celery, and green pepper. Cook, stirring occasionally, for 5 minutes or until vegetables are tender crisp.

2. Mix flour with broth in a shaker container, and stir in with all remaining ingredients. Bring soup to a boil, then reduce heat to simmer 15 more minutes.

Mulligatawny Soup (continued)

116 calories per serving
4 gm. fat, 8 gm. protein, 13 gm. carbohydrate,
0 cholesterol, 345 mg. sodium.

For exchange diets, count: 1 starch, 1 very lean meat.

Paella Shrimp Salad

Preparation time: 20 minutes

4 servings—2 cups each

1 1/2 cups no-added-salt vegetable broth
1 1/4 cups instant rice
1/8 teaspoon ground turmeric
1/4 teaspoon dried oregano
1/2 pound shrimp, cooked, peeled, and deveined
10-ounce package frozen peas, thawed and drained
1 ripe tomato, chopped
1/2 cup fat-free Italian dressing
1 teaspoon finely grated lemon rind
1 green onion, diced fine
fresh greens
garnish: lemon slices

1. Combine broth and rice in a microwave-safe dish, and cover. Cook on high power for 5 minutes. Remove cover, and add 2 large ice cubes to speed cooling.

2. Combine cooled rice with all remaining ingredients in a large salad bowl. Stir to blend, then chill until serving time. Arrange fresh greens on 4 salad plates, and divide salad among the 4 plates. Garnish with fresh lemon slices.

197 calories per serving
2 gm. fat, 18 gm. protein, 27 gm. carbohydrate,
87 mg. cholesterol, 591 mg. sodium.

For exchange diets, count: 1 starch,
2 vegetable, 2 very lean meat.

Pinto Bean Chili

Preparation time: 20 minutes

8 servings—1 1/2 cups each

1 teaspoon vegetable oil
1 large green pepper, washed, seeded and diced
1 large white onion, chopped fine
1/2 teaspoon minced garlic
1 fresh jalapeno pepper, seeded and chopped or 1 tablespoon dried
    hot peppers
24-ounce can stewed tomatoes
16-ounce can pinto beans, drained and rinsed
16-ounce can kidney beans, drained and rinsed
1 cup no-added-salt beef broth
2 tablespoons chili powder
2 teaspoons cumin
garnish: nonfat sour cream

1. In a large stock pot or Dutch oven sauté pepper, onion, garlic, and jalapeno in vegetable oil until vegetables are soft. Add all remaining ingredients and bring mixture to a boil. Reduce heat to a simmer for 10 minutes and serve with nonfat sour cream as a garnish on the side.

136 calories per serving
1 gm. fat, 7 gm. protein, 26 gm. carbohydrate,
0 cholesterol, 972 mg. sodium
(*to reduce sodium, use no-added-salt tomatoes*).

For exchange diets, count: 2 vegetables, 1 starch.

Potato and Ham Chowder

Preparation time: 10 minutes
Cooking time: 15 minutes

8 servings—1 1/2 cups each

2 (16-ounce) cans no-added-salt chicken broth
1 small onion, chopped fine
1 fresh carrot, washed and sliced thin
1 bay leaf
1/2 teaspoon dried thyme
1/2 teaspoon dried tarragon
2 (16-ounce) cans sliced potatoes, drained
16-ounce can whole kernel corn, drained
1 cup evaporated skim milk
1 tablespoon chopped pimiento
2 tablespoons chopped parsley
2 ounces lean ham, cut into thin strips

1. Combine all ingredients in order listed in a stockpot. Simmer over medium heat for 15 minutes or until carrots are done to desired tenderness. Reduce heat to low until serving time.

165 calories per serving
2 gm. fat, 8 gm. protein, 32 gm. carbohydrate,
5 mg. cholesterol, 154 mg. sodium.

For exchange diets, count: 1 1/2 starch, 1/2 skim milk.

Red Bean and Rice Supper Salad

Add a hot breadstick and a slice of cheese and this is a meal!

Preparation time: 20 minutes
8 servings—1 cup each

4 cups cooked rice
15-ounce can garbanzo beans, drained and rinsed
2 large fresh tomatoes, seeded and chopped
1 onion, chopped
1/4 cup chopped black olives

Dressing:
1/2 cup reduced-fat vinaigrette salad dressing
1/2 teaspoon dried basil
1/2 teaspoon dried thyme
1/2 teaspoon dried rosemary
1/2 teaspoon black pepper

1. In a large salad bowl, mix first five ingredients.

2. In a shaker container, mix ingredients for the dressing. Pour dressing over the salad; toss and serve.

208 calories per serving
2 gm. fat, 6 gm. protein, 43 gm. carbohydrate,
0 cholesterol, 242 mg. sodium.

For exchange diets, count: 2 starch, 2 vegetable.

Roasted Onion and Garlic Soup

A favorite of Dr. Mike Downey, who tasted it
at the Victoria Cottage in Decorah, Iowa.

Preparation time: 20 minutes
Roasting time: 45 minutes
Cooking time: 20 minutes

8 servings—1 cup each

3 large onions, unpeeled
8 large cloves garlic, unpeeled
2 tablespoons olive oil, divided
5 cups no-added-salt chicken or beef broth
1 1/2 teaspoons dried thyme
1 large potato, peeled and diced fine
garnish: minced fresh parsley or chives

1. Preheat oven to 375°.

2. Place onions and garlic in a baking dish. Sprinkle with 1 tablespoon
olive oil. Roast for 45 minutes.

3. Add 1 tablespoon of olive oil to a stockpot, and heat over medium
heat. Remove vegetables from the oven. Squeeze out soft garlic pulp
into the stockpot. Peel onions, and slice them into the stockpot. Sauté
onion and garlic in the oil for 3 minutes. Stir in broth, thyme, and diced
potato. Simmer for 15 minutes, then purée just until potatoes are
mashed. Serve; or chill and reheat for later service.

73 calories per serving
4 gm. fat, 2 gm. protein, 8 gm. carbohydrate,
0 cholesterol, 43 mg. sodium.

For exchange diets, count: 1/2 starch, 1 fat.

Salmon Pasta Salad with Cucumber and Dill

Preparation time: 20 minutes
Chilling time: 30 minutes

8 servings—2 cups each

8 ounces fettuccini, cooked as package directs, rinsed and drained
1 large carrot, peeled and shredded
1 large cucumber, peeled, seeded, and diced
2 ribs celery, diced fine
16-ounce can salmon, drained and flaked

Dressing:
  1/3 cup lemon juice
  1/2 cup reduced-fat mayonnaise
  1/2 cup fat-free sour cream
  3 teaspoons chicken-flavor low-sodium instant bouillon
  1 tablespoon Dijon-style mustard
  1 1/2 teaspoons dill weed

1. In a large salad bowl, combine the first five ingredients.

2. In a mixing bowl, blend ingredients for the dressing. Pour over the salad ingredients, and toss to mix. Cover and chill for at least 30 minutes or until serving time.

168 calories per serving
5 gm. fat, 16 gm. protein, 14 gm. carbohydrate,
43 mg. cholesterol, 268 mg. sodium.

For exchange diets, count: 1 starch, 2 very lean meat, 1/2 fat.

Spinach Salad with Canadian Bacon

Preparation time: 20 minutes

4 servings—2 cups each

Salad:
    1 pound spinach, washed and torn into bite-size pieces
    11-ounce can mandarin oranges, drained
    1 small red onion, sliced thin
    8 ounces Canadian bacon, cut into thin strips

Dressing:
    1 envelope dry honey mustard salad dressing mix
    1/4 cup cider vinegar
    2 tablespoons orange juice
    1/2 cup water

1. Combine salad ingredients in a large serving bowl.

2. Combine ingredients for the dressing in a shaker container, and shake to mix well. Pour dressing over the salad, and toss to coat.

182 calories per serving
5 gm. fat, 18 gm. protein, 20 gm. carbohydrate,
33 mg. cholesterol, 1,492 mg. sodium
(to reduce sodium, use half of salad dressing mix).

For exchange diets, count: 1 fruit, 1 vegetable, 2 lean meat.

Pork and Brown Rice Salad with Balsamic Vinaigrette

Preparation time: 15 minutes

4 servings—1 1/2 cups each

Salad:
    1/2 pound cooked pork, cut into thin strips
    2 cups cooked brown rice
    1 cup green grapes, cut in half
    1 cup fresh strawberries, sliced in half

Dressing:
    1/2 cup orange juice
    1 tablespoon vegetable oil
    2 tablespoons balsamic vinegar
    2 teaspoons apple juice concentrate
    1 teaspoon Dijon mustard

    fresh greens

1. Combine ingredients for the salad in a large serving bowl.

2. Combine ingredients for the dressing in a shaker container, and shake to mix. Pour dressing over salad; toss. Serve on a bed of crispy fresh greens.

304 calories per serving
8 gm. fat, 19 gm. protein, 39 gm. carbohydrate,
45 mg. cholesterol, 47 mg. sodium.

For exchange diets, count: 2 starch, 1/2 fruit, 2 lean meat.

Tex-Mex Corn Relish and Smoked Turkey Salad

Preparation time: 15 minutes

8 servings—1 1/2 cups each

1 cup instant rice
1 cup no-added-salt chicken broth
12-ounce jar corn relish, drained
2 cups diced smoked turkey breast
1/2 cup chunky salsa
garnish: fresh cilantro

1. Combine rice and broth in a microwave-safe dish. Cover and cook on high power for 4 minutes. Remove cover, and stir in 2 large ice cubes to speed cooling.

2. In a large salad bowl, combine cooled rice with next 3 ingredients. Stir to mix. Serve on chilled salad plates with chopped fresh cilantro as a garnish.

178 calories per serving
0 fat, 19 gm. protein, 25 gm. carbohydrate,
48 mg. cholesterol, 916 mg. sodium
*(to reduce sodium, use no-added-salt salsa
and fresh roasted turkey).*

For exchange diets, count: 1 starch,
1 vegetable, 2 very lean meat.

30-Minute Chicken Soup

Feel a cold coming on? This remedy is ready in a half hour.

Preparation time: 10 minutes
Cooking time: 20 minutes

4 servings—1 1/2 cups each

3 (14-ounce) cans chicken broth
9-ounce can diced cooked chicken
1/4 teaspoon salt
2 ribs celery, chopped
2 green onions, chopped
2 carrots, peeled and sliced thin
3 whole cloves
1/2 teaspoon nutmeg
2 teaspoons dried parsley
1 bay leaf
1 cup frozen peas
8 ounces fresh mushrooms, sliced thin
2 ounces noodles of choice, uncooked

1. Combine all ingredients except noodles in a large stockpot. Bring to a boil, reduce to simmer, and cook covered for at least 20 minutes. Add noodles during last 8 minutes of cooking time.

267 calories per serving
7 gm. fat, 26 gm. protein, 25 gm. carbohydrate,
56 mg. cholesterol, 357 mg. sodium.

For exchange diets, count: 1 starch,
2 1/2 lean meat, 2 vegetable.

Turkey Salad with Fruit and Rice

Preparation time: 20 minutes

4 servings—1 1/2 cups each

1 cup no-added-salt chicken broth
1 cup instant rice
16-ounce can diced peaches in juice
2 cups diced white meat turkey
2 ribs celery, diced fine

Dressing:
1 teaspoon vegetable oil
2 tablespoons cider vinegar
2 tablespoons pineapple or orange juice
1/2 teaspoon minced garlic
1/4 teaspoon cumin
1/8 teaspoon cinnamon
1/8 teaspoon cloves

1. Combine broth with instant rice in a microwave-safe container. Cover and cook on high power for 3 minutes. Uncover, and stir in 2 large ice cubes to speed cooling.

2. Drain peaches, reserving juice for another use. Toss turkey and celery with peaches in a large salad bowl. Add cooled rice.

3. Mix ingredients for the dressing together in a shaker container, then pour over the salad, and toss to coat. Serve with reduced-fat wheat crackers.

228 calories per serving
5 gm. fat, 27 gm. protein, 19 gm. carbohydrate,
73 mg. cholesterol, 118 mg. sodium.

For exchange diets, count: 3 very lean meat, 1/2 fruit, 1 starch.

Chapter Five

Salads

Broccoli, Bean, and Bowtie Pasta Salad

Preparation time: 15 minutes

8 servings—1 cup each

4 ounces bowtie pasta, cooked tender and drained
   (DO NOT OVERCOOK)
11-ounce can mandarin oranges, drained
15-ounce can garbanzo beans, drained and rinsed
1 large bunch fresh broccoli, washed, trimmed, and chopped
2 green onions, sliced thin

Dressing:
   1/4 cup white vinegar
   1/4 cup orange juice
   1 tablespoon vegetable oil
   1 teaspoon basil
   1 teaspoon oregano
   1/4 teaspoon minced garlic
   1/4 teaspoon pepper

1. In a large salad bowl, toss cooled pasta with mandarin oranges,and vegetables.

2. In a shaker container, combine ingredients for the dressing; shake to mix. Pour dressing over the salad. Serve immediately or cover and refrigerate until serving time.

113 calories per serving
0 fat, 5 gm. protein, 23 gm. carbohydrate,
0 cholesterol, 186 mg. sodium.

For exchange diets, count: 1 starch, 1 vegetable.

Caesar Salad Dressing

Preparation time: 10 minutes
Chilling time: 4 hours

16 servings—2 tablespoons each

2 cups fat-free mayonnaise or salad dressing
1 teaspoon dried basil
1 teaspoon minced garlic
1 teaspoon coarsely ground black pepper
1/2 cup freshly grated Parmesan cheese

1. Combine all ingredients in a 3 cup bowl that has a tight-fitting lid. Stir ingredients well. Refrigerate at least 4 hours before using with green salads.

40 calories per serving
2 gm. fat, 1 gm. protein, 6 gm. carbohydrate,
8 mg. cholesterol, 270 mg. sodium.

For exchange diets, count: 1/2 starch.

Citrus Salad with a Spicy Crunch

Preparation time: 20 minutes
Chilling time: 1 hour

12 servings—2/3 cup each

4 oranges, peeled and cut into small pieces
2 red grapefruit, peeled and cut into pieces
16-ounce can red kidney beans, drained well
4 ribs celery, sliced thin
1 green onion, sliced thin

Dressing:
1 tablespoon vegetable oil
1 tablespoon lemon juice
1/4 cup pineapple juice
1/4 teaspoon salt
1/2 teaspoon oregano

1. Combine fruits with kidney beans, celery, and onion in a large salad bowl.

2. In a shaker container, combine ingredients for dressing. Pour dressing over salad, and stir to mix. Refrigerate for an hour or until serving time.

87 calories per serving
1 gm. fat, 3 gm. protein, 17 gm. carbohydrate,
0 cholesterol, 200 mg. sodium.

For exchange diets, count: 1 fruit, 1/2 very lean meat.

Coconut Coleslaw

Preparation time: 15 minutes
Chilling time: 30 minutes

8 servings—1 cup each

1 pound shredded cabbage and carrots
8-ounce can crushed pineapple, drained
1/4 cup golden raisins
1/4 flaked coconut
1/3 cup nonfat mayonnaise

1. Combine all ingredients in a big salad bowl. Cover and chill for at least 30 minutes or until serving time.

95 calories per serving
4 gm. fat, 2 gm. protein, 16 gm. carbohydrate,
0 cholesterol, 141 mg. sodium.

For exchange diets, count: 1 fat, 1 vegetable, 1/2 fruit.

Copper Penny Salad

Preparation time: 15 minutes

8 servings—3/4 cup each

1 1/2 pounds carrots, cut into coins
1/2 green pepper, chopped fine
1 scallion, sliced fine

Dressing:
    8-ounce can no-added-salt tomato sauce
    1/4 cup vinegar
    sugar substitute equivalent to 2 tablespoons of sugar
    1 teaspoon prepared mustard
    1/2 teaspoon celery seed

1. Place sliced carrots and 1 tablespoon. water into microwave-safe 2-quart dish. Cover with plastic wrap and microwave on high for 3 minutes. Drain well.

2. Transfer carrots to a 2-quart salad bowl. Add green pepper and scallion.

3. Combine dressing ingredients in a shaker container and pour over vegetables, tossing to coat. This salad keeps well in the refrigerator for up to 4 days.

77 calories per serving
0 fat, 2 gm. protein, 14 gm. carbohydrate,
0 cholesterol, 71 mg. sodium.

For exchange diets, count: 1 starch.

Corn Relish with Pepper and Pimiento

Preparation time: 15 minutes
Chilling time: 30 minutes

12 servings—1/2 cup each

2 (1-pound) cans whole kernel corn, well drained
4 ribs celery, sliced diagonally
1 small red pepper, chopped
1/4 cup chopped pimiento

Dressing:
1/2 teaspoon dried chives
1/8 cup vegetable oil
1/4 cup vinegar
1 teaspoon Nutrasweet Spoonful sugar substitute
1/2 teaspoon salt
1/2 teaspoon paprika
1/2 teaspoon dry mustard
3 drops hot sauce

1. Mix drained corn with celery, pepper, and pimiento in a salad bowl.

2. In a shaker container, combine dressing ingredients. Pour over corn mixture. Cover and refrigerate for at least 30 minutes to allow flavors to blend.

99 calories per serving
3 gm. fat, 2 gm. protein, 17 gm. carbohydrate,
0 cholesterol, 113 mg. sodium.

For exchange diets, count: 1 starch, 1/2 fat.

Creamy Cucumber Salad

Preparation time: 15 minutes
Chilling time: 4 hours

8 servings—3/4 cup each

2 medium cucumbers, peeled and sliced thin
1 teaspoon dill weed
1 teaspoon salt
1/4 teaspoon black pepper
sugar substitute equivalent to 1 tablespoon of sugar
2 tablespoons red wine vinegar
2 green onions, diced
1 cup nonfat sour cream
8 cherry tomatoes, sliced in half

1. In a large salad bowl, combine all the ingredients except the tomatoes. Stir to blend, then cover and refrigerate at least 4 hours. Add tomatoes just before serving.

55 calories per serving
0 fat, 3 gm. protein, 12 gm. carbohydrate,
0 cholesterol, 48 mg. sodium.

For exchange diets, count: 2 vegetables.

Creamy Nonfat Coleslaw

Preparation time: 15 minutes
Chilling time: 1 hour

8 servings—3/4 cup each

1-pound bag of shredded cabbage
1 large green pepper, diced
2/3 cup nonfat mayonnaise
1/8 cup cider vinegar
1/2 teaspoon salt
1/2 teaspoon lemon juice
1/4 teaspoon black pepper
1 tablespoon Nutrasweet Spoonful sugar substitute

1. Combine shredded cabbage and diced pepper in a salad bowl.

2. In a small mixing bowl, combine remaining ingredients, and blend until smooth. Pour dressing over cabbage, and mix thoroughly. Serve immediately or chill for 1 hour for a better blend of flavors.

35 calories per serving
0 fat, 1 gm. protein, 7 gm. carbohydrate,
0 cholesterol, 282 mg. sodium.

For exchange diets, count: 1 vegetable.

Diet Mountain Dew Salad

Preparation time: 15 minutes
Chilling time: 2 hours

8 servings—3/4 cup each

6-ounce package sugar-free lemon flavored gelatin
2 cups boiling water
20-ounce can crushed pineapple in juice, drained and juice reserved
1 cup diet Mountain Dew

Topping:
    1 cup nonfat sour cream
    1 teaspoon lemon extract
    1/4 cup Equal Measure sugar substitute

1. In a large mixing bowl, dissolve gelatin in boiling water. Add diet Mountain Dew and reserved pineapple juice. Refrigerate this mixture for 30 minutes until thickened, but not set.

2. Fold in crushed pineapple, and transfer to an shallow 11" x 7" dish. Refrigerate 1 1/2 hours.

3. Combine ingredients for topping in a small bowl, and spread on top of salad. Cut and serve.

56 calories per serving
0 fat, 3 gm. protein, 12 gm. carbohydrate,
0 cholesterol, 46 mg. sodium.

For exchange diets, count: 1 fruit.

Eight-Minute Microwave Fruit Salad

Preparation time: 8 minutes

8 servings—1/2 cup each

3-ounce package sugar-free vanilla pudding
10-ounce can pineapple tidbits in juice
10-ounce can mandarin oranges in juice
2 fresh kiwi, peeled and sliced into coins
2 cups red grapes, washed

1. Drain juices from pineapple and oranges into a 1-cup glass measure. Add water to make 1 cup of liquid. Pour the liquid into a microwave-safe salad bowl.

2. Whisk in the pudding mix, then microwave on high power for 6 minutes, stopping to stir the mixture twice.

3. Add 4 large ice cubes to the mixture to speed cooling, and stir until they are dissolved.

4. Fold in pineapple, oranges, sliced kiwi, and grapes. Serve immediately or cover and refrigerate until serving time. This salad lasts very well in the refrigerator.

65 calories per serving
0 fat, 1 gm. protein, 16 gm. carbohydrate,
0 cholesterol, 52 mg. sodium.

For exchange diets, count: 1 fruit.

Fat-Free Creamy Italian Salad Dressing

Preparation time: 10 minutes
Chilling time: 4 hours

16 servings—2 tablespoons each

2 cups fat-free mayonnaise or salad dressing
2 tablespoons red wine vinegar
sugar substitute equivalent to 1 tablespoon sugar
2 teaspoons dried basil
2 teaspoons dried oregano
1/2 teaspoon minced garlic
1/2 teaspoon black pepper
1 teaspoon dried fennel

1. Combine all ingredients in a 3-cup bowl that has a tight-fitting lid.
Stir ingredients well. Refrigerate at least 4 hours before using with
green salads.

30 calories per serving
0 fat, 1 gm. protein, 6 gm. carbohydrate,
0 cholesterol, 240 mg. sodium.

For exchange diets, count: 1/2 fruit.

Fat-Free Onion and Dill Salad Dressing

Preparation time: 10 minutes
Chilling time: 4 hours

16 servings—2 tablespoons each

2 cups fat-free mayonnaise or salad dressing
1 tablespoon dill weed
1 teaspoon onion powder
1 tablespoon skim milk

1. Combine all ingredients in a 3 cup bowl that has a tight-fitting lid. Stir ingredients well. Refrigerate at least 4 hours before using with green salads.

30 calories per serving
0 fat, 1 gm. protein, 6 gm. carbohydrate,
0 cholesterol, 240 mg. sodium.

For exchange diets, count: 1/2 fruit.

Fat-Free Taco Salad Dressing

Preparation time: 10 minutes
Chilling time: 4 hours

16 servings—2 tablespoons each

2 cups fat-free mayonnaise or salad dressing
1 teaspoon chili powder
1/2 teaspoon ground cumin
1 teaspoon minced garlic
1/3 cup mild salsa
1/4 cup sun-dried tomatoes, chopped fine

1. Combine all ingredients in a 3-cup bowl that has a tight-fitting lid. Stir ingredients well. Refrigerate at least 4 hours before using with green salads.

30 calories per serving
0 fat, 1 gm. protein, 6 gm. carbohydrate,
0 cholesterol, 240 mg. sodium.

For exchange diets, count: 1/2 fruit.

15-Minute Potluck Vegetable Salad

Preparation time: 15 minutes

8 servings—3/4 cup each

4 ribs celery, chopped fine
1 large onion, chopped fine
20 ounces frozen mixed vegetables, thawed and drained

Dressing:
  1/2 cup cider vinegar
  1 tablespoon flour
  1 tablespoon prepared mustard
  1/2 teaspoon white pepper
  1/4 cup Equal Measure sugar substitute

1. In a large mixing bowl, combine chopped celery, onion, and thawed vegetables. If you need to thaw the vegetables in a hurry, run the plastic bag or box under warm tap water until you can feel the vegetables soften. Then drain.

2. In a small saucepan, whisk together the vinegar, flour, and mustard. Heat over medium heat to boiling; boil for 1 minute. Remove from heat and stir in pepper and sugar substitute. Add 1 ice cube to speed cooling of the dressing.

3. Pour dressing over the vegetables. Serve immediately, or cover and refrigerate for up to 1 week.

60 calories per serving
0 fat, 4 gm. protein, 10 gm. carbohydrate,
0 cholesterol, 31 mg. sodium.

For exchange diets, count: 2 vegetables

5-Layer Ribbon Salad

Preparation time: 2 hours

16 servings—1 square each

3-ounce package sugar-free lime gelatin
14-ounce can evaporated skim milk
3-ounce package sugar-free cherry gelatin
3-ounce package sugar-free lemon gelatin
3-ounce package sugar-free orange gelatin
3-ounce package sugar-free raspberry gelatin

1. In a 9" x 13" glass dish, dissolve lime gelatin in 1/2 cup of hot water. Stir in 1/2 cup of cold water and 1/2 cup of evaporated skim milk. Refrigerate 20 minutes until set.

2. In a glass bowl, dissolve cherry gelatin in 3/4 cup hot water. Stir in 3/4 cup cold water. Pour over first layer, and refrigerate for at least 20 minutes or until firm.

3. In same glass bowl, dissolve lemon gelatin in 1/2 cup hot water. Add 1/2 cup of cold water and 1/2 cup of evaporated skim milk. Pour over second layer, and refrigerate for at least 20 minutes or until firm.

4. In same glass bowl, dissolve orange gelatin in 3/4 cup hot water. Add 3/4 cup cold water, then pour over third layer. Refrigerate at least 20 minutes or until firm.

5. In same glass bowl, dissolve raspberry gelatin in 1/2 cup hot water. Stir in 1/2 cup cold water and 1/2 cup evaporated skim milk; pour over fourth layer. Refrigerate at least 20 minutes or until firm.

6. Cut salad into 16 servings, and serve on lettuce-lined salad plates for a special occasion.

21 calories per serving
0 fat, 2 gm. protein, 3 gm. carbohydrate,
0 cholesterol, 41 mg. sodium.

For exchange diets, count: 1 vegetable.

Five-Minute Five-Cup Salad

Preparation time: 5 minutes

8 servings—generous 1/2 cup each

8-ounce can pineapple tidbits, in juice, drained well
11-ounce can mandarin oranges in juice, drained well
8-ounce can chunky mixed fruit in juice, drained well
1 cup fresh grapes, cut in half
1 cup reduced-fat sour cream
2 tablespoons Equal Measure sugar substitute
garnish: 1/4 cup flaked coconut

1. Combine drained fruits with grapes, sour cream, and sugar substitute in a salad bowl. Stir to mix. Smooth out the top of the salad, and use a spatula to remove dressing from the sides of the bowl. Sprinkle with coconut; cover and serve immediately or chill until serving time.

86 calories per serving
0 fat, 3 gm. protein, 20 gm. carbohydrate,
0 cholesterol, 44 mg. sodium.

For exchange diets, count: 1 1/2 fruit.

Frosted Raspberry Salad

Preparation time: 20 minutes

12 servings—1/12 pan each

2 (3-ounce) packages sugar-free raspberry gelatin
1 cup hot water
16-ounce bag frozen whole raspberries
20-ounce can crushed pineapple, drained
1 pint nonfat sour cream
2 teaspoons almond extract
1 tablespoon Nutrasweet Spoonful sugar substitute
1/4 cup chopped pecans

1. Dissolve gelatin in the hot water in a large mixing bowl. Fold in berries and pineapple. Pour half of this mixture into an 11" x 7" glass dish. Refrigerate for 2 hours.

2. Mix sour cream with almond extract and sugar substitute. Spread 1 1/2 cups of the sour cream mixture over the gelatin, then cover with remaining gelatin. Refrigerate 2 more hours.

3. Spread remaining 1/2 cup sour cream mixture on top. Garnish with chopped pecans. Cut in squares, and serve on a lettuce leaf.

94 calories per serving
2 gm. fat, 3 gm. protein, 16 gm. carbohydrate,
0 cholesterol, 54 mg. sodium.

For exchange diets, count: 1/2 fat, 1 fruit.

German Potato Salad

The sweet and sour taste of this dish makes it a favorite.

Preparation time: 20 minutes
Cooking time: 20 minutes—Baking time: 30 minutes

8 servings—3/4 cup each

4 large potatoes, peeled and sliced
2 strips bacon, diced fine

Sauce:
1 teaspoon dry mustard
1/2 cup no-added-salt chicken broth
1 egg, beaten
1/2 tablespoon flour
1/2 teaspoon salt
1/2 cup cider vinegar
1/2 cup Equal Measure sugar substitute

1. Preheat oven to 350°.

2. Boil or steam the potato slices until tender. Cook bacon in a small skillet until crisp; drain.

3. Meanwhile, in a medium saucepan, combine mustard, broth, egg, flour, salt, and vinegar. Use an egg beater to whip the mixture to a smooth consistency. Then cook over medium heat for 5 minutes, stirring constantly until the mixture thickens. Stir in sugar substitute.

4. Layer potatoes with bacon in a large baking dish. Pour sauce over the potatoes, and bake uncovered for 30 minutes.

88 calories per serving
2 gm. fat, 3 gm. protein, 15 gm. carbohydrate,
29 mg. cholesterol, 122 mg. sodium.

For exchange diets, count: 1 starch.

Jicama and Fruit Salad

Preparation time: 15 minutes

4 servings—1 cup each

16-ounce can chunky mixed fruit in juice
1 small jicama, peeled and cut into julienne strips
2 green onions, sliced

Dressing:
2 tablespoons lime juice
1/2 teaspoon chili powder
1 tablespoon fresh cilantro, minced (may substitute parsley)
dash of salt
1 teaspoon vegetable oil

1. Drain the fruit, saving the juice for another use. Combine with strips of jicama and green onions in a salad bowl.

2. Combine ingredients for the dressing in a shaker container and shake to mix. Pour dressing over the salad, and toss. Serve with a plain sandwich meal.

84 calories per serving
1 gm. fat, 2 gm. protein, 18 gm. carbohydrate,
0 cholesterol, 9 mg. sodium.

For exchange diets, count: 1 starch.

Lemon Pepper and Parmesan Dressing

Preparation time: 15 minutes

8 servings—2 tablespoons each

1/4 cup olive oil
1 tablespoon fresh lemon juice
2 teaspoons lemon pepper seasoning
2 teaspoons Dijon-style mustard
1/2 teaspoon minced garlic
1/4 cup rice-wine vinegar
1/4 cup grated Parmesan cheese

1. Combine all ingredients in a shaker container, and shake to mix. Serve with tossed green salads or your favorite main dish salads.

70 calories per serving
7 gm. fat, 1 gm. protein, 0 carbohydrate,
2 mg. cholesterol, 60 mg. sodium.

For exchange diets, count: 1 1/2 fat.

Low-Fat Potato Salad

Preparation time: 15 minutes
Cooking time: 25 minutes
Chilling time: 1 hour

16 servings—3/4 cup each

6 large potatoes, peeled, boiled, and chopped
3 eggs, hardboiled and sliced
4 ribs celery, thinly sliced
1 yellow onion, diced

Dressing:
　　1 cup nonfat sour cream
　　1/2 cup reduced-fat mayonnaise
　　3 tablespoons vinegar
　　1/2 teaspoon salt
　　1/4 teaspoon pepper
　　1 tablespoon dill pickle relish

1. Combine cooked potatoes and eggs with celery and onion in a salad bowl.

2. In a small mixing bowl, combine dressing ingredients. Pour dressing over potatoes, and fold to blend. Refrigerate for at least 1 hour or until ready to serve.

100 calories per serving
3 gm. fat, 3 gm. protein, 14 gm. carbohydrate,
42 mg. cholesterol, 129 mg. sodium.

For exchange diets, count: 1/2 fat, 1 starch.

Marinated Black Bean Salad

Preparation time: 15 minutes
Chilling time: 30 minutes

8 servings—3/4 cup each

2 (16-ounce) cans black beans, drained well
1 red pepper, seeded and diced
1 yellow pepper, seeded and diced
1 small red onion, diced

Dressing:
   1/2 teaspoon salt
   1/4 cup red wine vinegar
   1/4 teaspoon minced garlic
   1/4 teaspoon ground cumin
   1 teaspoon hot pepper sauce
   1 tablespoon olive oil
   2 tablespoons prune juice, grape juice, or apple juice

1. Combine drained beans with diced vegetables in a large salad bowl.

2. Mix ingredients for the dressing together in a shaker container and blend. Pour dressing over beans. Stir and refrigerate at least 30 minutes to allow flavors to blend.

183 calories per serving
2 gm. fat, 8 gm. protein, 34 gm. carbohydrate,
0 cholesterol, 73 mg. sodium.

For exchange diets, count: 2 starch, 1 vegetable.

One-Bowl Lemon-Dressed Fruit Medley

Preparation time: 15 minutes
Chilling time: 2 hours

8 servings—3/4 cup each

3-ounce package sugar-free lemon gelatin
1 cup boiling water
6 large ice cubes
3 ounces frozen orange juice concentrate
6 ounces pineapple juice
4 cups assorted fresh fruits, cut into chunks (pineapple tidbits, sliced
green grapes, and diced apples make a nice combination)

1. In a large salad bowl, combine gelatin and boiling water. Stir until gelatin is fully dissolved. Stir in ice cubes, orange juice concentrate, and pineapple juice.

2. Add 4 cups of assorted fresh fruits, and refrigerate for at least 2 hours or until ready to serve. This combination lasts in the refrigerator for 2 days.

83 calories per serving
0 fat, 0 protein, 22 gm. carbohydrate,
0 cholesterol, 1 mg. sodium.

For exchange diets, count: 1 1/2 fruit.

Orange Pineapple Salad

Preparation time: 15 minutes
Chilling time: 2 hours

4 servings—3/4 cup each

3-ounce package sugar-free orange gelatin
1 cup boiling water
1 cup orange juice
1 tablespoon white vinegar
1 large carrot, cleaned and grated
1/4 cup crushed pineapple, drained well

1. In a medium mixing bowl, pour boiling water over gelatin; stir to mix well. Stir in remaining ingredients, then pour into a small square shallow dish. Cut in squares and serve on a lettuce leaf. Refrigerate at least 2 hours.

42 calories per serving
0 fat, 1 gm. protein, 10 gm. carbohydrate,
0 cholesterol, 8 mg. sodium.

For exchange diets, count: 1/2 fruit.

Pea Salad

Preparation time: 15 minutes
Chilling time: up to 24 hours

8 servings—3/4 cup each

16-ounce bag frozen green peas; thawed and drained well
2 ounces reduced-fat cheddar cheese, cubed
2 egg whites, chopped
2 ribs celery, chopped fine
1 very small white onion, chopped

Dressing:
1/3 cup reduced-fat mayonnaise
1/4 teaspoon salt
1/4 teaspoon Tabasco sauce
1/8 teaspoon pepper

1. In a medium salad bowl, combine peas, cheese, egg whites, celery, and onion.

2. In a small mixing bowl, combine remaining ingredients for dressing.

3. Fold dressing into the peas. Serve immediately, or refrigerate for up to 24 hours. Garnish with paprika.

112 calories per serving
5 gm. fat, 6 gm. protein, 10 gm. carbohydrate,
5 mg. cholesterol, 264 mg. sodium.

For exchange diets, count: 1 fat, 1 vegetable, 1/2 starch.

Picnic Pasta Salad

There's no mayonnaise to worry about in this summer favorite.

Preparation time: 20 minutes; Chilling time: 30 minutes
8 servings—1 1/2 cups each

8 ounces seashell macaroni
1 tablespoon vegetable oil
1/4 cup Equal Measure sugar substitute
1/4 cup cider vinegar
1/4 cup wine vinegar
1/4 cup water
1 tablespoon prepared mustard
1/4 teaspoon black pepper
2 ounces pimientos, drained
2 small cucumbers, peeled, cut into fourths lengthwise,
   and diced thin
2 green onions, thinly sliced
garnish: cherry tomatoes

1. Cook pasta according to package directions, taking care not to over-cook. Drain well, rinse with cold water, and drain again.

2. Place sugar substitute, vinegars, water, mustard, pepper, and pimiento in a blender container. Process at low speed for 10 seconds or just until flecks of pimiento can be seen.

3. Combine cooked pasta with cucumbers and onions in a large salad bowl. Pour dressing over all. Cover and chill at least 30 minutes. At picnic time, garnish the salad with halved cherry tomatoes.

80 calories per serving
2 gm. fat, 2 gm. protein, 14 gm. carbohydrate,
0 cholesterol, 27 mg. sodium.

For exchange diets, count: 1 starch.

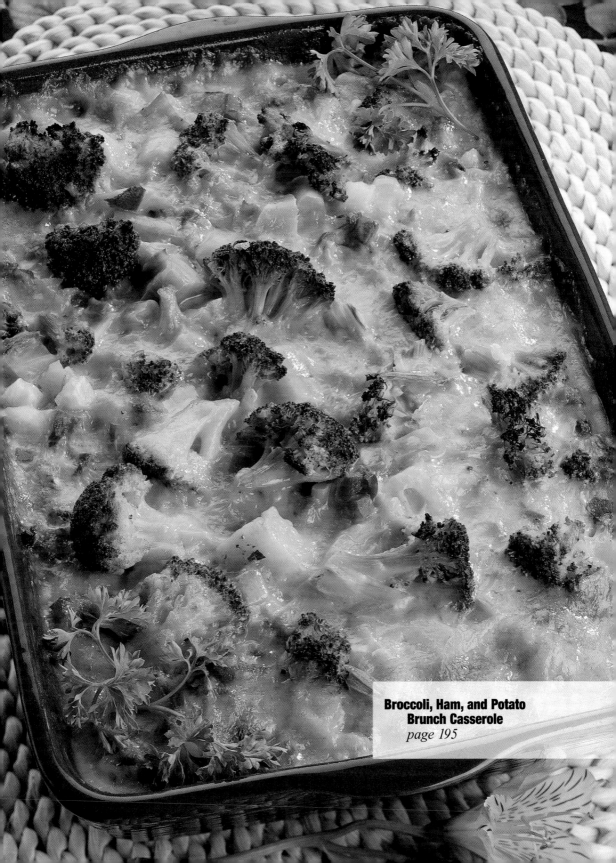

**Broccoli, Ham, and Potato
Brunch Casserole**
page 195

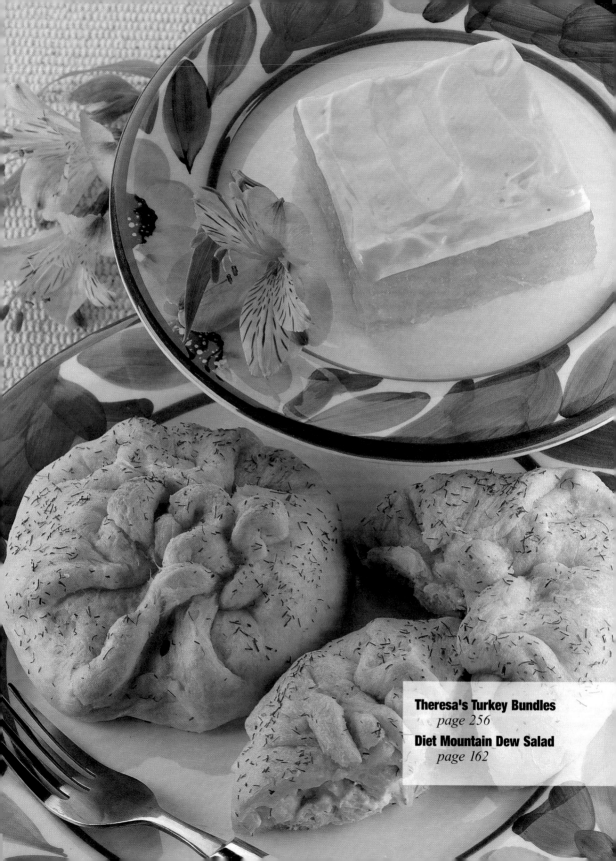

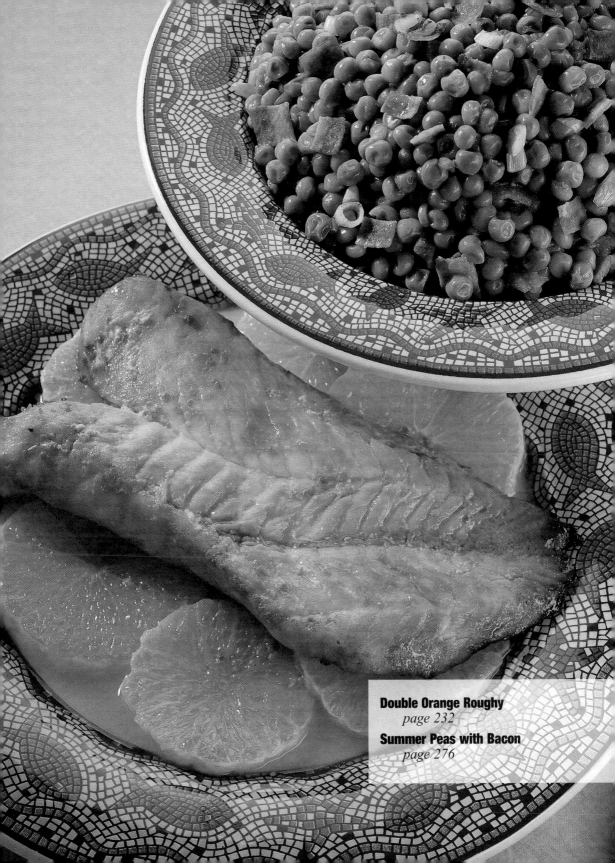

Double Orange Roughy
page 232

Summer Peas with Bacon
page 276

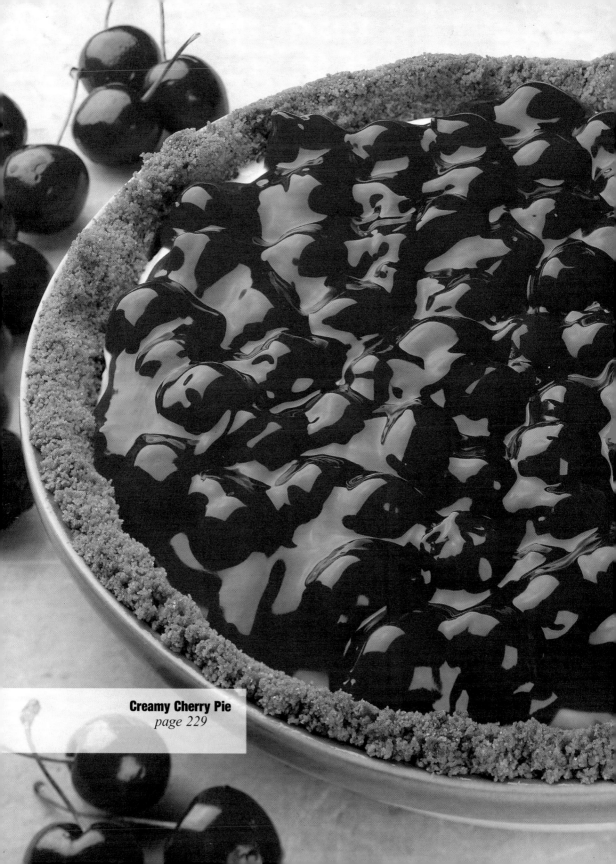

Creamy Cherry Pie
page 229

Pineapple Lover's Salad

Preparation time: 15 minutes
Chilling time: 2 hours

12 servings—1/2 cup each

20 ounces crushed pineapple, not drained
6 ounces fat-free cream cheese, softened
8 ounces sugar-free vanilla yogurt
20 ounces pineapple chunks, drained
8 ounces reduced-fat whipped topping
garnish: fresh mint

1. Combine crushed pineapple and pineapple juice with softened cream cheese and yogurt in a large salad bowl. Blend until smooth.

2. Gently fold in drained pineapple chunks and whipped topping. Chill at least 2 hours or until ready to serve.

118 calories per serving
3 gm. fat, 3 gm. protein, 21 gm. carbohydrate,
1 mg. cholesterol, 57 mg. sodium.

For exchange diets, count: 1/2 skim milk, 1 fruit.

Raspberry Vinaigrette Salad Dressing

Preparation time: 10 minutes

8 servings—1 1/2 tablespoons each

1/2 cup raspberry juice
1 teaspoon dried tarragon
1 tablespoon olive oil
1/4 cup red wine vinegar
1 teaspoon Dijon-style mustard
1/2 teaspoon salt

1. Combine all ingredients in a shaker container. Mix well and refrigerate for use with green salads.

23 calories per serving
2 gm. fat, 0 protein, 2 gm. carbohydrate,
0 cholesterol, 80 mg. sodium.

For exchange diets, count: 1/2 fat.

Red and Green Grape Salad

Preparation time: 10 minutes
Chilling time: 30 minutes

8 servings—2/3 cup each

2 cups red grapes, washed and halved
2 cups green grapes, washed and halved
1 cup nonfat sour cream
1/4 cup Equal Measure sugar substitute
1/4 cup coarsely chopped pecans

1. Mix all ingredients together in a salad bowl. Chill at least 30 minutes or until serving time.

147 calories per serving
5 gm. fat, 3 gm. protein, 27 gm. carbohydrate,
0 cholesterol, 40 mg. sodium.

For exchange diets, count: 1 fat, 1 1/2 fruit.

Sauerkraut Confetti Salad

Preparation time: 15 minutes
Chilling time: 2 hours

8 servings—1 cup each

16-ounce can sauerkraut
1 rib celery, finely chopped
1 green onion, diced
3 large carrots, shredded
1/3 cup Nutrasweet Spoonfuls sugar substitute
1/4 cup vinegar

1. Drain sauerkraut, and reserve 1/4 cup of the liquid. Snip the kraut into bite-size pieces. Combine kraut with celery, onion and carrot in a medium salad bowl.

2. Combine reserved 1/4 cup of sauerkraut juice, sugar substitute, and vinegar in a small bowl; stir to mix well. Toss dressing with vegetables to coat. Chill for at least 2 hours or up to 3 days.

60 calories per serving
0 fat, 0 protein, 15 gm. carbohydrate,
0 cholesterol, 389 mg. sodium.

For exchange diets, count: 1 vegetable, 1/2 fruit.

Spicy Marinated Pear Salad

Preparation time: 15 minutes
Chilling time: 30 minutes

4 servings—2 cups each

16-ounce can pear slices in juice
1 red onion, sliced thin
1 tablespoon lime juice
1/4 teaspoon minced garlic
1/4 teaspoon ground coriander
dash of salt
1/4 teaspoon pepper
4 cups shredded lettuce or spinach

1. Drain pears well, reserving juice for another use. Toss pears with sliced onion in a salad bowl. Combine lime juice, garlic, coriander, salt, and pepper in a shaker container; mix well. Pour dressing over the pears and onions, and toss to coat. Refrigerate at least 30 minutes.

2. Divide shredded lettuce among 4 chilled salad plates. Spoon marinated pears and onions over the lettuce, and serve with a plain grilled meat.

76 calories per serving
0 fat, 4 gm. protein, 17 gm. carbohydrate,
0 cholesterol, 19 mg. sodium.

For exchange diets, count: 1 fruit, 1 vegetable.

Spinach Salad with Creamy Raspberry Vinaigrette

Preparation time: 15 minutes

4 servings—2 cups each

1 pound fresh spinach, torn into bite-size pieces
1 red onion, thinly sliced and separated into rings
1 cup fresh raspberries

Dressing:
    1/2 cup nonfat plain yogurt
    2 tablespoons raspberry vinegar
        or 1 teaspoon raspberry juice plus 5 teaspoons vinegar
    1/4 teaspoon salt
    1/2 teaspoon Dijon mustard
    1/4 teaspoon minced garlic
    1 teaspoon dried parsley
    1 teaspoon vegetable oil

1. Combine spinach, onion, and berries in a large salad bowl. Chill if desired.

2. In a small mixing bowl, combine ingredients for the dressing. Chill if preparing ahead of serving. Pour dressing over salad at serving time and toss.

77 calories per serving
2 gm. fat, 2 gm. protein, 15 gm. carbohydrate,
0 cholesterol, 185 mg. sodium.

For exchange diets, count: 2 vegetable, 1/2 fat.

Strawberry Banana Salad

Preparation time: 10 minutes
Chilling time: 2 hours

4 servings—3/4 cup each

1 package plain gelatin (such as Knox)
1/2 cup water
1 cup sugar-free strawberry yogurt
10-ounce package frozen strawberries, thawed
2 large bananas, peeled and sliced

1. In a 1-quart glass microwave-safe salad bowl, stir gelatin into water. Microwave on high power for 45 seconds, just until gelatin is dissolved. Stir in yogurt, strawberries, and sliced bananas. Chill for at least 2 hours.

86 calories per serving
0 fat, 2 gm. protein, 20 gm. carbohydrate,
0 cholesterol, 165 mg. sodium.

For exchange diets, count: 1 1/2 fruit.

Sugar-Free Perfection Salad

Preparation time: 10 minutes
Chilling time: 2 hours

8 servings—3/4 cup each

2 (3-ounce) packages sugar-free lemon gelatin
2 cups boiling water
1 cup cold water
1/3 cup vinegar
2 tablespoons lemon juice
2 cups shredded cabbage
1/2 cup shredded carrots
1/2 cup chopped celery
1/2 cup chopped green pepper

1. Combine lemon gelatin and 2 cups boiling water in a mixing bowl. Stir to completely dissolve gelatin. Stir in 1 cup cold water, vinegar, and lemon juice. Chill mixture for 30 minutes.

2. Fold in vegetables, and turn mixture into a 6-cup mold or an 8" square dish. Chill until set, at least 1 1/2 hours. Serve on lettuce-lined salad plate. Garnish the salad with reduced-fat mayonnaise at serving time.

32 calories per serving
0 fat, 1 gm. protein, 7 gm. carbohydrate,
0 cholesterol, 32 mg. sodium.

For exchange diets, count: 1 vegetable.

Sweet and Sour Three-Bean Salad

Preparation time: 15 minutes

12 servings—2/3 cup each

16-ounce can green beans, well drained
16-ounce can red kidney beans, well drained
16-ounce can wax beans, well-drained
1 large white onion, chopped fine

Dressing:
    1 tablespoon vegetable oil
    3/4 cup vinegar
    1/4 cup Nutrasweet Spoonful sugar substitute
    1 teaspoon salt
    1/2 teaspoon black pepper

1. In a salad bowl, mix drained beans with onion.

2. In a shaker container, mix all remaining ingredients. Pour dressing over beans, and stir carefully. Serve immediately or refrigerate until ready to serve. This salad lasts 3 days and is a never-fail quick side dish for soups and sandwiches.

105 calories per serving
1 gm. fat, 6 gm. protein, 18 gm. carbohydrate,
0 cholesterol, 210 mg. sodium.

For exchange diets, count: 1 starch, 1 vegetable.

Tangy Marinated Onion Salad

Preparation time: 15 minutes
Chilling time: 30 minutes

8 servings—3/4 cup each

1 large sweet onion, thinly sliced and separated into rings
4 large ripe tomatoes, sliced
1 cucumber, peeled and sliced thin

Dressing:
2 tablespoons vegetable oil
1/4 cup red wine vinegar
1 teaspoon Dijon mustard
1/2 teaspoon salt
1/4 black pepper
sugar substitute equivalent to 1/2 teaspoon sugar
1 teaspoon dried basil

1. Place half of the onions in a large shallow salad bowl. Layer the tomato and cucumber slices over the onion. Top with remaining onion rings.

2. In a shaker container, combine all remaining ingredients and then pour over the vegetables. Cover and chill for at least 30 minutes or until ready to serve. This salad keeps for 2 days.

67 calories per serving
3 gm. fat, 2 gm. protein, 8 gm. carbohydrate,
0 cholesterol, 141 mg. sodium.

For exchange diets, count: 1 vegetable, 1 fat.

Waldorf Salad

Preparation time: 15 minutes

8 servings—3/4 cup each

1 pound green seedless grapes, washed and halved
2 large red apples, cored and cubed
1/2 cup seedless raisins
1/4 cup chopped walnuts
2 ribs celery, diced fine
1/2 cup nonfat mayonnaise
1/2 cup nonfat, sugar-free vanilla yogurt
3-4 deep green outer leaves from romaine lettuce, chopped

1. Combine fruits in a large salad bowl.

2. In a small glass cup, stir together mayonnaise and yogurt. Pour over fruits, and stir to mix. Serve this salad on a bed of chopped greens.

149 calories per serving
4 gm. fat, 3 gm. protein, 28 gm. carbohydrate,
0 cholesterol, 207 mg. sodium.

For exchange diets, count: 1 fruit, 1/2 skim milk, 1 fat.

Zesty Carrot and Raisin Salad

Preparation time: 15 minutes

4 servings—3/4 cup each

2 cups shredded carrots
1/2 cup minced green pepper
1/3 cup raisins
1 tablespoon minced onion
1/2 cup crushed pineapple in juice

Dressing:
2 tablespoons cider vinegar
1 tablespoon vegetable oil
sugar substitute equivalent to 2 teaspoons of sugar
1/4 teaspoon celery seeds
1/4 teaspoon dry mustard

1. In a medium salad bowl, combine first 5 ingredients.

2. In a shaker container, combine remaining ingredients. Pour dressing over salad just before serving.

119 calories per serving
4 gm. fat, 2 gm. protein, 209 gm. carbohydrate,
0 cholesterol, 154 mg. sodium.

For exchange diets, count: 1 fruit, 1 vegetable, 1 fat.

Chapter Six

Low-Meat
and
No-Meat
Entrées

Bean and Bacon Casserole

Hands on preparation time: 10 minutes
Cooking time: Slow cooker method—4-6 hours
Microwave method—20 minutes

16 servings—2/3 cup each

1/4 pound Canadian bacon, cut into 1/2-inch chunks
1 medium onion, chopped fine
28-ounce can pork and beans with tomato sauce
15-ounce can butter beans, drained
15-ounce can pinto beans, drained
1/4 cup apple juice concentrate
1/3 cup catsup
2 tablespoons vinegar
1 teaspoon dry mustard
1 teaspoon maple flavoring

1. Combine all ingredients in a slow cooker and cook on low for 4 to 6 hours. If you are in a hurry, mix all ingredients together in a 3-quart casserole dish; cover and cook in the microwave on 70% power for 18 to 20 minutes, stirring twice during cooking.

151 calories per serving
4 gm. fat, 9 gm. protein, 21 gm. carbohydrate,
6 mg. cholesterol, 175 mg. sodium.

For exchange diets, count: 1 very lean meat, 1 1/2 starch.

Broccoli, Ham, and Potato Brunch Casserole

Preparation time: 15 minutes
Baking time: 45 minutes

8 servings—1 1/2 cups each

nonstick cooking spray
2 cups frozen chopped broccoli
4 ounces lean ham, diced
3 cups frozen hash browns
1 can reduced-fat cheddar cheese soup
1 1/2 soup cans skim milk
4 ounces reduced-fat American cheese, shredded

1. Preheat oven to 375°.

2. Spray an 11" x 7" baking dish with cooking spray. Layer broccoli, ham, and hash browns in the pan. Mix cheddar cheese soup with milk in a small bowl, and pour over the other ingredients. Bake for 30 minutes.

3. Sprinkle with shredded cheese, and bake an additional 15 minutes.

135 calories per serving
4 gm. fat, 10 gm. protein, 18 gm. carbohydrate,
13 mg. cholesterol, 617 mg. sodium.

For exchange diets, count: 1 starch, 1 lean meat.

Broccoli and Brown Rice Deep Skillet Dinner

Preparation time: 20 minutes
Cooking time: 10 minutes

4 servings—2 cups each

1 skinless, boneless chicken breast, diced
1/2 teaspoon minced garlic
1 1/2 cups no-added-salt chicken broth
1 small head of broccoli, broken into florets
1 red pepper, cut into thin strips
1 yellow squash, sliced thin
1/4 teaspoon black pepper
1 1/2 cups instant brown rice, dry
1 ounce freshly grated Parmesan cheese

1. In a deep skillet, heat chicken, garlic, broth, broccoli, red pepper, and squash to boiling. Stir in pepper and brown rice, and reduce heat to a simmer. Simmer uncovered for 5 minutes. Sprinkle Parmesan cheese on top, and serve.

139 calories per serving
2 gm. fat, 9 gm. protein, 21 gm. carbohydrate,
13 mg. cholesterol, 86 mg. sodium.

For exchange diets, count: 1 very lean meat,
1 starch, 1 vegetable.

Cheesy Potato and Ham Casserole

Preparation time: 10 minutes
Cooking time: slow cooker method—4 hours
Microwave method—20 minutes

8 servings—1 1/2 cups each

1 pound frozen hash browns or 4 large potatoes, peeled and cubed
1/4 cup chopped onion
1 cup low-fat buttermilk
1/2 cup soft cheddar cheese spread
10-ounce can reduced-fat cream of chicken soup
8 ounces lean ham, chopped

1. Mix all ingredients together in a slow cooker and cook for 4 hours on medium heat.

2. If you're in a hurry, mix all ingredients except ham in a 3-quart microwave dish, and cook in the microwave on 70% power for 12 minutes. Stop cooking at 4 and 8 minutes to stir well. At 12 minutes, stir in ham, then cook on high power for 2 more minutes.

153 calories per serving
6 gm. fat, 11 gm. protein, 18 gm. carbohydrate,
29 mg. cholesterol, 817 mg. sodium
(*to reduce sodium, choose turkey instead of ham*).

For exchange diets, count: 1 starch, 1 1/2 lean meat.

Chicken à la King

Preparation time: 20 minutes
Cooking time: 15 minutes

4 servings—1 1/2 cup each

1 teaspoon reduced-fat margarine
1 green onion, chopped fine
1/2 green pepper, chopped fine
1/2 cup flour
3 1/2 cups no-added-salt chicken broth
2 whole boneless, skinless cooked chicken breasts, diced
8-ounce can sliced mushrooms, drained
1/2 teaspoon salt
1/4 teaspoon white pepper
1 egg or 1/4 cup liquid egg substitute
3/4 cup skim milk
1/4 cup chopped pimiento
4 large or 8 small baking powder biscuits

1. In a deep skillet, melt margarine. Add the onion and green pepper and cook over medium heat for 3 minutes or until the vegetables are soft. Remove vegetables from the skillet and set aside. Add the flour to the pan, and pour in chicken broth. Stir with a whisk, and cook over medium heat for 4 minutes or until the mixture is thick. Fold in diced cooked chicken, drained mushrooms, sautéed onion, and pepper, and seasonings. Continue cooking over low heat.

2. In a small bowl, combine the egg with the skim milk. Whisk this into the chicken mixture, and cook for 5 minutes. Fold in pimiento, and serve over baking powder biscuits.

171 calories per serving
3 gm. fat, 17 gm. protein, 21 gm. carbohydrate,
23 mg. cholesterol, 279 mg. sodium.

For exchange diets, count: 2 very lean meat, 1 starch, 1 vegetable.

Chicken and Broccoli Pot Pie

Preparation time: 15 minutes
Baking time: 30 minutes

8 servings—1 slice each

nonstick cooking spray
1 bunch fresh broccoli, broken into florets
1 cup cooked diced chicken or turkey
1 medium yellow onion, chopped
4 ounces reduced-fat cheddar cheese, shredded
1 1/3 cups skim milk
3 eggs or 3/4 cup liquid egg substitute
3/4 cup reduced-fat baking mix (such as Bisquick Light)
1/4 teaspoon salt
1/4 teaspoon pepper
1/2 teaspoon curry powder
optional garnish: red pepper flakes

1. Preheat oven to 400°.

2. Spray a 10" pie pan with cooking spray. Layer first four ingredients in the pan.

3. In a blender container, combine remaining ingredients. Blend on medium speed for 30 seconds or until mixture is smooth. Pour egg mixture into the pan. If desired, sprinkle red pepper flakes on the egg mixture. Bake for 25 to 30 minutes until firm. Allow pie to sit at room temperature for 10 minutes before slicing. This recipe may be assembled a day ahead and refrigerated overnight. Increase baking time to 35 minutes for chilled mixture.

226 calories per serving
6 gm. fat, 21 gm. protein, 22 gm. carbohydrate,
107 mg. cholesterol (27 mg. with egg substitute),
570 mg. sodium.

For exchange diets, count: 1 starch, 1 vegetable,
3 very lean meat.

Chicken Chow Mein

Preparation time: 20 minutes
Baking time: 30 minutes

4 servings—2 cups each

nonstick cooking spray
1 teaspoon reduced-fat margarine
2 ribs celery, finely chopped
1 medium onion, chopped fine
10-ounce can reduced-fat cream of chicken soup
4-ounce can sliced mushrooms, drained well
2 tablespoons cashews, chopped
2 boneless, skinless cooked chicken breast halves, diced
12-ounce can chow mein noodles

1. Preheat oven to 400°. Spray a casserole dish with cooking spray.

2. In a deep skillet, melt margarine. Add celery and onion, and cook until vegetables are soft. Add soup, mushrooms, cashews, and diced chicken; and stir to mix.

3. Transfer the mixture to casserole dish. Bake for 20 minutes. Fold two-thirds of the noodles into the chicken, and return to the oven for 10 more minutes. Sprinkle the remaining noodles on the casserole just before serving.

248 calories per serving
12 gm. fat, 16 gm. protein, 19 gm. carbohydrate,
28 mg. cholesterol, 367 mg. sodium.

For exchange diets, count: 2 lean meat,
1 starch, 1 vegetable, 1/2 fat.

Feta-Flavored White Beans and Rice

Preparation time: 20 minutes
Cooking time: 15 minutes

8 servings—1 cup each

1 teaspoon olive oil
1 yellow onion, chopped fine
1 teaspoon minced garlic
1/2 pound fresh spinach, washed, stems removed, and torn into small
    pieces
16-ounce can chunky tomatoes
1 cup instant rice
1 cup no-added-salt chicken broth
16-ounce can white beans, drained
2 teaspoons dried mint leaves
    (or 2 tablespoons fresh mint, chopped fine)
1 teaspoon dried rosemary, crushed
1 tablespoon red wine vinegar
1 tablespoon sherry
1/2 teaspoon salt
1/2 teaspoon black pepper
4 ounces feta cheese, crumbled

1. Measure oil into a Dutch oven and heat over medium heat. Add onion, garlic, and spinach and saute for 4 minutes. Add tomatoes, rice, and broth, and bring mixture to a boil. Reduce heat to simmer, and cook for 5 minutes. Add all remaining ingredients and heat through. Transfer rice and beans to a serving dish or serve directly onto dinner plates. Garnish with crumbled feta cheese.

117 calories per serving
1 gm. fat, 7 gm. protein, 21 gm. carbohydrate,
0 cholesterol, 255 mg. sodium.

For exchange diets, count: 1 1/2 starch.

Layered Italian Zucchini Casserole

Preparation time: 20 minutes
Cooking time: Conventional oven method—45 minutes
Microwave method—20 minutes

4 servings—1 1/2 cups each

1/2 pound lean ground beef, browned and drained
1 onion, chopped
1 green pepper, chopped
4 ounces fresh mushrooms, sliced thin
1/2 teaspoon olive oil
8 ounces no-added-salt tomato sauce
1/2 teaspoon garlic powder
1/2 teaspoon fennel
1/4 teaspoon black pepper
1 teaspoon basil
1 teaspoon oregano
2 ounces part-skim mozzarella cheese, shredded
2/3 cup nonfat cottage cheese
4 small zucchini, peeled and sliced thin lengthwise
1/3 cup grated Parmesan cheese
nonstick cooking spray

1. Preheat oven to 375° (if using the conventional oven).

2. In a medium skillet, brown meat; drain well. In same skillet, sauté chopped onion, pepper, and mushrooms in olive oil until soft. Stir in drained meat, tomato sauce, garlic powder, fennel, pepper, basil, and oregano.

3. In a small mixing bowl, combine mozzarella cheese and cottage cheese.

4. Spray an 11" x 7" casserole dish with cooking spray. Layer meat sauce, zucchini, and cheese mixture twice. Sprinkle Parmesan cheese

over the last meat layer. Bake in the oven for 45 minutes or cook in the microwave for 20 minutes. This casserole can be assembled and refrigerated or frozen for later baking.

216 calories per serving
4 gm. fat, 23 gm. protein, 22 gm. carbohydrate,
37 mg. cholesterol, 421 mg. sodium.

For exchange diets, count: 2 vegetable,
1 skim milk, 2 very lean meat

Ranch-Style Beans

Preparation time: 20 minutes
Cooking time: 2-4 hours

8 servings—1 cup each

16-ounce can dark red kidney beans, drained
24-ounce can pinto beans, drained
1 large onion, diced
1/4 cup grape or apple juice concentrate
1 tablespoon prepared mustard
14-ounce can chunky tomatoes, undrained
1 tablespoon cider vinegar
4 ounces Canadian bacon, diced fine

1. Combine all ingredients in a slow cooker. Cook on high power for 2 to 4 hours.

175 calories per serving
2 gm. fat, 12 gm. protein, 29 gm. carbohydrate,
8 mg. cholesterol, 744 mg. sodium
(to reduce sodium, use no-added-salt tomatoes).

For exchange diets, count: 1 starch, 1 very lean meat, 1 fruit.

Red Beans and Rice in One Skillet

Preparation time: 15 minutes
Cooking time: 20 minutes

8 servings—1 cup each

1/2 pound reduced-fat spicy pork sausage
1 large onion, chopped fine
1 large green pepper, cored, seeded, and diced
2 ribs celery, chopped
1/2 teaspoon minced garlic
16-ounce can kidney beans, drained
14-ounce can chunky tomatoes
1/2 cup red wine
1/2 cup water
1 cup instant rice
1 teaspoon rosemary leaves
1 teaspoon thyme
1/2 teaspoon salt
1/2 teaspoon pepper
1 teaspoon hot pepper sauce

1. In a large deep skillet, brown pork sausage with onion, pepper, celery, and garlic. Drain pork and vegetables well, and return them to the skillet. Add all remaining ingredients, and cook over medium heat for 10 minutes until rice is fluffy.

148 calories per serving
2 gm. fat, 12 gm. protein, 18 gm. carbohydrate,
22 mg. cholesterol, 329 mg. sodium.

For exchange diets, count: 1 starch,
1 vegetable, 1 very lean meat.

Sausage-Stuffed Peppers

Preparation time: 15 minutes
Baking time: 45 minutes

8 servings—1 pepper each

8 large fresh peppers, choose green, red, or yellow

Stuffing:
 1/2 pound reduced-fat spicy pork or turkey sausage
 1 rib celery, chopped fine
 1 small onion, chopped fine
 1 teaspoon thyme
 1 teaspoon black pepper
 2 cups corn bread stuffing mix
 10-ounce can reduced-fat condensed cream of chicken soup

1. Preheat oven to 400°.

2. Wash peppers, cut the tops off and remove the seeds and membranes, then set aside.

3. In a large skillet, brown the sausage with the celery and onion for 6 minutes or until the sausage is no longer pink. Stir in the remaining ingredients.

4. Stuff the peppers with the cornbread mixture, then place peppers in a baking dish. Cover and bake for 45 minutes; remove the cover during last 15 minutes of baking.

246 calories per serving
10 gm. fat, 10 gm. protein, 24 gm. carbohydrate,
24 mg. cholesterol, 915 mg. sodium
(*to reduce sodium, use plain croutons instead of stuffing mix*).

For exchange diets, count: 1 1/2 starch, 1 vegetable, 1 lean meat, 1 fat.

Shepherd's Pie

Preparation time: 15 minutes
Baking time: 30 minutes

8 servings—1 cup each

nonstick cooking spray
1/2 pound lean ground beef, browned and drained
1 tablespoon dried onion or 1 small onion, diced fine
13-ounce can reduced-fat cream of mushroom soup
1 tablespoon soy sauce
16-ounce can kitchen cut green beans, drained
2 cups leftover mashed potatoes
    or 2 cups prepared instant mashed potatoes
1 ounce reduced-fat cheddar cheese, shredded

1. Preheat oven to 400°. Spray an 8" square casserole dish with cooking spray.

2. Combine browned hamburger with onion, soup, and soy sauce in the prepared dish. Layer drained beans on top of the meat. Spread mashed potatoes over the top, and sprinkle with cheese. Bake for 30 minutes.

182 calories per serving
9 gm. fat, 11 gm. protein, 15 gm. carbohydrate,
34 mg. cholesterol, 400 mg. sodium
(to reduce sodium, use no-added-salt green beans).

For exchange diets, count: 1 starch, 1 lean meat, 1 fat.

Show-off Tamale Pie

This is a showy entrée for Mexican food lovers.

Preparation time: 20 minutes
Baking time: 25 minutes

8 servings—1 slice each

1/2 pound lean ground beef
1 tablespoon chili powder
2 teaspoons cumin
16-ounce can black beans, rinsed and drained
14-ounce can chunky Mexican-flavored tomatoes
2 ounces reduced-fat Monterey Jack cheese
1 cup nonfat sour cream
2 green onions, sliced thin

Crust:
8-ounce package corn muffin mix
2 ounces reduced-fat Monterey Jack cheese, shredded
1 cup nonfat sour cream
1/4 cup green chilies, drained
nonstick cooking spray

1. Preheat oven to 400°.

2. In a large nonstick skillet over medium heat, brown ground beef with chili power and cumin for 5 minutes or until beef is no longer pink. Drain meat well.

3. Add beans and tomatoes and heat to boiling; then reduce heat to simmer.

4. Meanwhile in a mixing bowl, combine all ingredients for the crust; stirring just until moist. Spray an 11" x 7" casserole dish with cooking

spray. Spoon two-thirds of the muffin mixture into the dish, spreading it over the bottom and up the sides. Spoon beef and bean mixture over the batter. Then dollop remaining muffin batter around the outside of the dish, spreading it around the outside edge and leaving a small open circle in the middle. Sprinkle the cheese on top of the batter and bake for 25 minutes.

5. When the pie is done, dollop the sour cream into the open circle and sprinkle with green onions. Allow the pie to sit for 5 minutes, then slice and serve.

228 calories per serving
8 gm. fat, 10 gm. protein, 26 gm. carbohydrate,
27 mg. cholesterol, 382 mg. sodium.

For exchange diets, count: 1 1/2 starch,
1 vegetable, 1 lean meat, 1/2 fat.

Sloppy Joe Pizza

Preparation time: 15 minutes
Baking time: 15 minutes

8 servings—1 slice each

1/2 pound lean ground beef
1 large green pepper, seeded and chopped
2 green onions, chopped fine
16-ounce can whole kernel corn, drained
2/3 cup barbecue sauce
12-inch prepared Italian bread shell (substitute your favorite pizza
    crust mix if you can't get a prepared bread shell)
4 ounces reduced-fat Cheddar cheese, shredded

1. Preheat oven to 425°.

2. In a large skillet, brown ground beef, green pepper, and onion for 5 minutes or until meat is no longer pink. Drain meat well. Then return meat to the pan, stir in corn and barbecue sauce, and heat to boiling.

3. Place bread shell on a large baking sheet and spread beef mixture over the shell. Sprinkle with cheese, and bake for 15 minutes.

339 calories per serving
10 gm. fat, 19 gm. protein, 43 gm. carbohydrate,
31 mg. cholesterol, 645 mg. sodium.

For exchange diets, count: 2 lean meat,
2 1/2 starch, 1 vegetable.

Smoked Corn-Stuffed Zucchini

Preparation time: 15 minutes
Baking time: 20 minutes

4 servings—2 stuffed shells each

4 medium zucchini, about 6 inches long

Filling:
    15-ounce can black beans, drained and rinsed
    11-ounce can Mexican-style corn, drained
    4-ounce can chopped green chilies, drained
    1/4 teaspoon liquid smoke
    1/2 teaspoon ground cumin
    2 ounces reduced-fat Monterey Jack cheese, shredded

1. Preheat oven to 400°.

2. Wash zucchini. then cut in half lengthwise. Remove most of the center with seeds, leaving a minimum of 1/4 to 1/2 inch of rind.

3. Combine the ingredients for the filling in a mixing bowl, then stuff the 8 zucchini halves. Place in a baking dish, and bake for 20 minutes or until the zucchini shells are bright green and the cheese is melted.

227 calories per serving
3 gm. fat, 12 gm. protein, 40 gm. carbohydrate,
0 cholesterol, 554 mg. sodium.

For exchange diets, count: 1 lean meat, 2 starch, 1 vegetable.

Stove Top Turkey and Noodles

Preparation time: 20 minutes

4 servings—1 1/2 cups each

4 ounces dry bowtie pasta, or wide ribbon pasta
2 tablespoons dry ranch salad dressing mix
1/2 cup skim milk
1/4 cup nonfat mayonnaise
2 cups frozen sugar snap peas, thawed
2 cups cubed cooked turkey

1. Cook pasta according to package directions. Drain well and return to the pan.

2. Meanwhile, combine salad dressing mix with milk and mayonnaise in a small bowl. Fold salad dressing mixture, peas, and turkey into drained pasta. Cook for 10 minutes over medium heat until the peas are cooked to desired doneness and the mixture is bubbly.

155 calories per serving
3 gm. fat, 16 gm. protein, 16 gm. carbohydrate,
43 mg. cholesterol, 315 mg. sodium.

For exchange diets, count: 2 very lean meat, 1 starch.

Sweet and Sour Shrimp

Preparation time: 20 minutes

8 servings—1 1/4 cups each

20-ounce can pineapple chunks in juice, drained and juice reserved
3/4 cup no-added-salt chicken broth
1/4 cup orange juice
1/4 cup vinegar
2 tablespoons brown sugar
   or 2 tablespoons Sugar Twin brown sugar substitute
3 tablespoons cornstarch
3 tablespoons reduced sodium soy sauce
1/4 teaspoon ground ginger
1/2 pound medium shrimp, peeled and deveined
8-ounce can sliced water chestnuts, drained
1 green bell pepper, cut into chunks
2 cups fresh snap peas or 6 ounces frozen snap peas, thawed

1. In a large skillet, combine reserved pineapple juice, chicken broth, orange juice, vinegar, sugar or sugar substitute, cornstarch, soy sauce, and ginger. Cook over medium heat until thickened. Add shrimp, and cook 3 minutes. Add all remaining ingredients, and heat through. Serve with cooked rice.

184 calories per serving
2 gm. fat, 10 gm. protein, 35 gm. carbohydrate,
44 mg. cholesterol, 442 mg. sodium.

For exchange diets, count: 1 vegetable,
2 fruit, 1 very lean meat.

Three-Way Lasagna

Vary this recipe by choosing Meat Lovers, Seafood,
or Veggie Lasagna!

Preparation time: 15 minutes
Baking time: 1 hour, 15 minutes

8 servings—1 slice each

nonstick cooking spray
24-ounce jar spaghetti sauce
2/3 cup water or red wine
1 pound lasagna noodles
4 ounces mozzarella cheese

Cheese layer:
    1 pint nonfat ricotta cheese
    1 whole egg
    1 teaspoon pepper
    1 teaspoon dried parsley
    1/4 cup finely grated Parmesan cheese
    2 ounces part-skim mozzarella cheese, shredded

Choose from these fillings:

Meat Lovers:
    1/2 pound reduced-fat spicy Italian sausage, browned and drained

Seafood:
    1/2 pound crab meat

Veggie:
    3 cups finely diced vegetables (peppers, onions, mushrooms, carrots
    are a good combination)

1. Preheat oven to 375°. Spray an 11" x 7" pan with cooking spray.

2. Pour about 1 cup of sauce over the bottom of the pan. Add water or wine and tilt the pan to mix. Then place one layer of noodles over the sauce. Spread half of the cheese mixture over the noodles, then top with another layer of noodles. Then spread your choice of filling over the noodles. Add another cup of sauce. Layer again with noodles, then remaining cheese mixture, and the last cup of sauce. Cover and bake for 1 hour. Remove cover, sprinkle with 4 ounces shredded mozzarella and bake 15 more minutes. Remove from the oven, allow the lasagna to sit for 10 minutes, then slice and serve.

Meat Lovers: 343 calories per serving
14 gm. fat, 20 gm. protein, 51 gm. carbohydrate,
51 mg. cholesterol, 35 mg. sodium.
For exchange diets, count: 2 starch,
1 vegetable, 2 lean meat, 1 fat.

Seafood: 297 calories per serving
8 gm. fat, 20 gm. protein, 41 gm. carbohydrate,
34 mg. cholesterol, 331 mg. sodium.
For exchange diets, count: 2 starch,
2 lean meat, 1 vegetable.

Veggie: 306 calories per serving
8 gm. fat, 18 gm. protein, 40 gm. carbohydrate,
34 mg. cholesterol, 195 mg. sodium.
For exchange diets, count: 2 vegetable,
2 starch, 1 1/2 lean meat.

Chapter Seven

Meat, Fish, *and* Poultry Entrées

All-Purpose Marinade

This recipe makes enough for four different plain meat meals, and can be stored in the refrigerator for up to 1 month.

Preparation time: 10 minutes
Marinating time: 30 minutes or up to overnight

2 cups—1/2 cup marinade for 4 different meals

4 cloves garlic, minced, or 1 teaspoon minced garlic
1/4 cup apple juice concentrate
2 teaspoons ground ginger
1/4 cup olive oil
1/2 cup cider vinegar
1 cup reduced-sodium soy sauce

1. Combine ingredients for marinade in a shaker container. Use 1/2 cup marinade to cover 4 servings of: white fish fillets, skinless boneless chicken breasts, sirloin steaks, or pork chops.

2. Place meat in a shallow container, pour on 1/2 cup marinade, cover, and place in the refrigerator for at least 30 minutes or up to overnight before grilling or broiling to desired doneness. Discard marinade after use.

11 calories per 2-tablespoon serving
3 gm. fat, 2 gm. protein, 3 gm. carbohydrate,
0 cholesterol, 972 mg. sodium
(High sodium alert).

For exchange diets, count: as a free food.

Baked Ham with Pear Glaze

Preparation time: 15 minutes
Baking time: 30 minutes

8 servings—4 ounces each

2 pounds precooked 97% lean ham

Glaze:
16-ounce can pear halves in juice (do not drain)
1 teaspoon vegetable oil
1 small onion, finely chopped
1/2 teaspoon minced garlic
1 teaspoon paprika
1/2 teaspoon dried oregano
dash of salt

1. Preheat oven to 300°.

2. Place ham in a baking dish.

3. Combine ingredients for the glaze in a blender container and purée smooth. Pour glaze over the ham, and bake uncovered for 30 minutes, just to heat through.

191 calories per serving
7 gm. fat, 24 gm. protein, 7 gm. carbohydrate,
60 mg. cholesterol, 1,365 mg. sodium
(High sodium alert).

For exchange diets, count: 1/2 fruit, 3 lean meat.

Black-Eyed Peas and Pork

Preparation time: 20 minutes
Cooking time: 20 minutes

4 servings—1 1/2 cups each

1/2 pound lean ground pork
1/2 teaspoon thyme
1 small onion, chopped fine
1 green pepper, chopped fine
16-ounce can black eyed peas, drained
14-ounce can chunky tomatoes
1/4 teaspoon salt
1/4 teaspoon black pepper

1. Brown pork with thyme, onion, and green pepper in a large skillet. Drain off any fat. Add all remaining ingredients and cook over medium heat for 10 minutes. Serve over hot rice.

231 calories per serving
3 gm. fat, 23 gm. protein, 26 gm. carbohydrate,
43 mg. cholesterol, 283 mg. sodium.

For exchange diets, count: 3 very lean meat,
2 vegetable, 1 starch.

Broiled Salmon with Chives

Preparation time: 10 minutes
Cooking time: Broiler method—20 minutes
Microwave method—6 minutes

4 servings—4 ounces each

nonstick cooking spray
1 pound salmon steaks, thawed (may substitute halibut, orange
   roughy or cod)
1 tablespoon fresh chopped chives
1/4 teaspoon pepper
1/4 teaspoon marjoram
1/2 fresh lemon

1. Place salmon steaks on baking sheet that has been sprayed with cooking spray. Sprinkle chives, pepper, and marjoram over fish. Squeeze fresh lemon juice over the spices. Broil under medium heat for 20 minutes or until salmon flakes with a fork.

2. If you prefer to use the microwave, cook uncovered for 6 minutes.

206 calories per serving
12 gm. fat, 23 gm. protein, 0 carbohydrate,
67 mg. cholesterol, 66 mg. sodium.

For exchange diets, count: 4 lean meat.

Chicken and Vegetable Skillet Meal

Preparation time: 15 minutes
Cooking time: 15 minutes

8 servings—1 1/4 cup each

13-ounce can no-added-salt chicken broth
2 tablespoons cornstarch
2 tablespoons reduced-sodium soy sauce
1/2 teaspoon ground ginger
1 teaspoon canola oil
1/2 teaspoon minced garlic
2 (3-ounce) boneless skinless chicken breasts, cut into strips
4 cups assorted fresh vegetables of choice
    (broccoli, carrots, snap peas, mushrooms, and pepper
    make a nice combination)
2 cups cooked rice

1. In a small mixing bowl, combine broth, cornstarch, soy sauce, and ginger. Stir until smooth, then set aside.

2. In a large skillet, heat oil over medium heat. Add garlic and chicken strips. Cook over medium heat for 8 minutes, stirring chicken occasionally. Add vegetables, and continue cooking over medium heat for 3 more minutes. Pour in broth and cornstarch mixture, and heat to boiling. Continue cooking for 2 minutes. Fold in rice, and serve.

158 calories per serving
2 gm. fat, 10 gm. protein, 25 gm. carbohydrate,
17 mg. cholesterol, 308 mg. sodium.

For exchange diets, count: 1 starch, 1 vegetable, 1 lean meat.

Chicken Breasts with Peach Salsa

Preparation time: 15 minutes
Baking time: 30 minutes

4 servings—4 to 5 ounces each

Salsa:
  2 medium peaches, peeled, seeded, and diced
  1 red pepper, seeded and diced
  1 green onion, diced fine
  2 tablespoons lemon juice
  1 teaspoon dried mint
  1 teaspoon vegetable oil
  3/4 teaspoon ground ginger
  1/4 teaspoon ground red pepper

  nonstick cooking spray
  4 skinless boneless chicken breast halves

1. Preheat oven to 400°.

2. Combine ingredients for the salsa in a small bowl.

3. Arrange chicken breasts in a baking dish that has been sprayed with cooking spray. Pour salsa over the chicken, and bake for 30 minutes.

152 calories per serving
5 gm. fat, 18 gm. protein, 9 gm. carbohydrate,
44 mg. cholesterol, 38 mg. sodium.

For exchange diets, count: 1/2 fruit, 2 lean meat.

Chicken Creole in 15 Minutes

Preparation time: 15 minutes
Cooking time: 15 minutes

4 servings—1 chicken breast
+ 1/2 cup vegetable + 3/4 cup rice each

1 1/2 cups instant rice
1 1/2 cups water

Creole:
    4 medium skinless boneless chicken breast halves, cut into chunks
    14-ounce can chunky tomatoes
    1 cup chili sauce
    1 large green pepper, chopped
    2 ribs celery, chopped
    1 small onion, chopped fine
    1/2 teaspoon minced garlic
    1/2 teaspoon hot sauce
    1 teaspoon dried basil
    1/4 teaspoon crushed red pepper
    1 teaspoon dried parsley

1. Combine rice with water in a microwave-safe dish. Cover and cook on high power for 4 minutes.

2. Meanwhile, cook chicken in a large skillet over medium-high heat for 4 minutes or until it is no longer pink. Add all remaining ingredients. Bring to a boil, then reduce heat to simmer for 10 minutes or until vegetables are tender crisp. Serve creole over rice.

223 calories per serving
4 gm. fat, 21 gm. protein, 27 gm. carbohydrate,
48 mg. cholesterol, 472 mg. sodium.

For exchange diets, count: 3 lean meat, 1 starch, 2 vegetable.

Chicken Pot Pie

Preparation time: 20 minutes
Baking time: 15 minutes

4 servings—1/4 pie each

1 teaspoon soft margarine
1 small onion, chopped fine
10-ounce package frozen mixed vegetables
11-ounce can white meat chicken, drained
3/4 cup water
1/2 cup skim milk
1-ounce package chicken gravy mix
nonstick cooking spray
4-ounce package refrigerated buttermilk biscuits

1. Preheat oven to 425°.

2. In a large saucepan, melt margarine. Add onion, and cook for 3 minutes, stirring often. Add vegetables, chicken, water, milk, and gravy mix; bring mixture to a boil.

3. Spray a 2-quart baking dish with cooking spray. Spoon chicken mixture into the baking dish. Cut biscuits in half and arrange over the top. Bake for 15 minutes.

248 calories per serving
8 gm. fat, 22 gm. protein, 22 gm. carbohydrate,
0 cholesterol, 658 mg. sodium.

For exchange diets, count: 1 vegetable,
1 starch, 2 1/2 lean meat.

Chinese Pork and Bamboo Shoots

Preparation time: 25 minutes
Chilling time: 30 minutes
Cooking time: 20 minutes

8 servings—3/4 cup each

1 pound boneless pork loin, well trimmed
2 teaspoons soy sauce
1 teaspoon cornstarch
8 large mushrooms, sliced
2 eggs, slightly beaten, or 1/2 cup liquid egg substitute
1/2 teaspoon salt
2 teaspoons vegetable oil
8-ounce can bamboo shoots, drained and cut into 1/4-inch strips
1/4 cup water
3 tablespoons soy sauce
1 clove garlic, minced
sugar substitute equivalent to 1 teaspoon of sugar
1 tablespoon cold water
1 teaspoon cornstarch
4 scallions, cut diagonally into 1/4-inch pieces

1. Cut pork into slices. Stack slices, then cut lengthwise into strips.

2. Mix 2 teaspoons soy sauce and 1 teaspoon cornstarch in glass bowl; stir in pork. Cover and refrigerate 30 minutes.

3. Mix eggs and salt. Cook eggs until firm, turning once. Remove eggs from pan and cut into thin strips.

4. Heat oil in wok or skillet until hot. Cook and stir pork in oil until no longer pink. Add mushrooms, bamboo shoots, 1/4 cup water, 3 tablespoons soy sauce, garlic, and sugar substitute. Heat to boiling. Mix 1 tablespoon water and 1 teaspoon cornstarch. Add to pork mixture, and

stir until thick. Add egg strips and scallions and stir for 30 seconds. Serve over hot rice.

151 calories per serving
5 gm. fat, 20 gm. protein, 4 gm. carbohydrate,
105 mg. cholesterol with eggs (52 mg. cholesterol
with egg substitute), 658 mg. sodium.
(to reduce sodium, use reduced-sodium soy sauce).

For exchange diets, count: 2 1/2 lean meat, 1 vegetable.

Classic Barbecue Sauce for Chicken or Red Meats

Preparation time: 15 minutes

4 servings—3 tablespoons each

1/2 cup tomato ketchup
2 tablespoons prepared mustard
1 clove garlic, minced (or 1/4 teaspoon garlic powder)
1 tablespoon Worcestershire sauce
1 tablespoon dry red wine
1 tablespoon frozen orange juice concentrate

1. Combine all ingredients. Spread over grilled red meat or chicken when meat is almost done. Grill 2 minutes; turn and coat the other side. Grill 2 more minutes, and serve.

40 calories per serving
0 fat, 1 gm. protein, 10 gm. carbohydrate,
0 cholesterol, 532 mg. sodium.

For exchange diets, count: 1 fruit.

Corned Beef and Kraut Casserole

Preparation time: 20 minutes
Baking time: 30 minutes

4 servings—1 square each

nonstick cooking spray
16-ounce can sauerkraut
1/2 pound lean corned beef, cooked and shredded
3/4 cup reduced-fat baking mix
1 cup skim milk
1/2 cup nonfat mayonnaise
2 eggs or 1/2 cup liquid egg substitute
1 ounce reduced-fat Swiss cheese, shredded

1. Preheat oven to 400°.

2. Spray an 11" x 7" casserole dish with cooking spray. Spread the sauerkraut over the bottom of the pan. Top with the shredded corned beef.

3. In a medium mixing bowl, combine baking mix, milk, mayonnaise, and eggs. Stir until no lumps remain. Pour the mixture over the kraut and corned beef. Bake for 20 minutes. Top the casserole with cheese, then bake 5 to 10 more minutes.

380 calories per serving
10 gm. fat, 29 gm. protein, 39 gm. carbohydrate,
59 mg. cholesterol, 1,743 mg. sodium
(high sodium alert: I have had no success in
reducing sodium in this recipe).

For exchange diets, count: 2 starch, 2 vegetable, 3 lean meat.

Cornflake Chicken or Fish

Preparation time: 10 minutes
Baking time: chicken—45 minutes
fish—20 minutes

4 servings—4 ounces each

2 egg whites, whipped
1 1/2 cup evaporated skim milk
1 teaspoon poultry seasoning
3 cups crushed cornflakes
1 pound chicken, skinned, in pieces, or 1 pound frozen fish fillets

1. Preheat oven to 400°.

2. Combine egg whites, milk, and seasoning in a mixing bowl. Whip for 2 minutes.

3. Meanwhile, crush cornflakes in a plastic bag. Dip chicken or fish in milk and egg mixture, then shake in cornflakes, and place on a baking sheet. Bake chicken for 35 to 45 minutes. For fish, reduce time to 15 to 20 minutes.

215 calories per serving
9 gm. fat, 25 gm. protein, 5 gm. carbohydrate,
66 mg. cholesterol, 230 mg. sodium.

For exchange diets, count: 3 lean meat, 1/2 starch.

Crunchy Beef Burritos

Preparation time: 20 minutes
Baking time: 14 minutes

8 servings—1 burrito each

Sauce:
8 ounces no-added-salt tomato sauce
1/4 teaspoon garlic powder
1/2 teaspoon cumin
1/8 teaspoon cayenne powder (optional)
1/2 teaspoon dried jalapeño peppers (optional)
1 tablespoon lemon juice
1 tablespoon raisins (this sweetens the sauce)

1 pound lean ground beef, cooked and drained
8 (10-inch) flour tortillas
4 ounces part-skim American cheese, shredded
1/4 cup chopped scallions

1. Preheat oven to 350°.

2. Mix the sauce ingredients together. Pour over the drained beef, and stir to mix.

3. Place 1/2 cup beef mixture in each tortilla; fold and place seam side down on a baking sheet. Top with cheese and scallions. Bake uncovered for 15 minutes. Serve with lettuce and tomatoes. These burritos freeze well on sheets or in baking dishes.

212 calories per serving
6 gm. fat, 18 gm. protein, 20 gm. carbohydrate,
57 mg. cholesterol, 180 mg. sodium.

For exchange diets, count: 1 starch, 1 vegetable, 2 lean meat.

Double Orange Roughy

Preparation time: 10 minutes
Marinating time: 15 minutes
Broiling time: 10 minutes

4 servings—4 ounces each

4 (4-ounce) orange roughy fillets, thawed
1/3 cup reduced-sodium soy sauce
1 teaspoon ground ginger
2 teaspoons grated orange peel
1/2 teaspoon vegetable oil
1/2 teaspoon minced garlic
1/2 cup orange juice
1 seedless orange, peeled and sliced thin
1 tablespoon sesame seeds

1. Place thawed fillets in a shallow glass dish. Sprinkle with soy sauce, ginger, orange peel, oil, and garlic, turning to coat. Allow fillets to marinate at least 15 minutes.

2. Drain fish, and broil under low heat for 5 minutes per side.

3. Meanwhile, in a skillet, heat orange juice over medium heat. Add orange slices and sesame seeds. Heat through, then transfer orange mixture to a serving platter. Place broiled fillets on the oranges, and serve.

164 calories per serving
3 gm. fat, 24 gm. protein, 10 gm. carbohydrate,
29 mg. cholesterol, 825 mg. sodium
(*to reduce sodium, use less soy sauce*).

For exchange diets, count: 1 fruit, 3 very lean meat.

Fat-Free Tartar Sauce for Baked Fish

Preparation time: 5 minutes

8 servings—1/4 cup each

1 cup plain yogurt
1 cup fat-free mayonnaise
1/4 cup finely chopped dill pickle
1 tablespoon dried parsley
2 tablespoons finely chopped pimiento
2 teaspoons dried onion
1/4 teaspoon curry powder

1. Combine all ingredients in a jar. Stir to mix. Refrigerate for use with baked or grilled whitefish fillets.

44 calories per serving
0 fat, 2 gm. protein, 9 gm. carbohydrate,
2 mg. cholesterol, 470 mg. sodium.

For exchange diets, count: 1/2 starch.

Five-Minute Roast Beef and Salsa Sandwiches

Preparation time: 5 minutes
Baking time: 30 minutes

4 servings—1 sandwich each

1 teaspoon chili powder
1/2 teaspoon ground cumin
1/4 teaspoon salt
1/4 teaspoon ground red pepper
1/2 pound cooked roast beef, sliced thin
1/2 cup chunky salsa
4 white sourdough rolls
1 cup finely chopped lettuce

1. Sprinkle seasonings in the bottom of a skillet. Add roast beef, and heat through over medium heat for 2 minutes, stirring. Add salsa and cook for 3 more minutes. Serve on sliced sourdough rolls with chopped lettuce.

304 calories per serving
5 gm. fat, 26 gm. protein, 38 gm. carbohydrate,
39 mg. cholesterol, 1,404 mg. sodium
(*to reduce sodium, use reduced-sodium salsa*).

For exchange diets, count: 2 starch, 2 vegetable, 3 very lean meat.

Garlic and Hot Pepper Marinade

Preparation time: 10 minutes
Marinating time: at least 30 minutes

8 servings—1 1/2 tablespoons each

2 tablespoons vegetable oil
1/3 cup lemon juice
2 tablespoons chopped jalapeño peppers
1 tablespoon chicken-flavor low-sodium instant bouillon
1 teaspoon ground ginger
1/2 teaspoon minced garlic
2 teaspoons dried thyme leaves
1/2 cup water
1/2 cup vegetable broth

1. Combine all ingredients in a shaker container. Refrigerate for up to 3 months. Use with pork chops, chicken or turkey breast fillets, or with fajita cuts of meat.

2. Marinate meat in a shallow covered container in the refrigerator for at least 30 minutes. Always discard marinade after use. Use half the batch (about 3/4 cup) with 4 pork chops.

35 calories per serving
4 gm. fat, 0 protein, 1 gm. carbohydrate,
0 cholesterol, 60 mg. sodium.

For exchange diets, count: 1 fat.

Grilled Italian Steak Sandwiches

Preparation time: 15 minutes
Marinating time: at least 15 minutes

4 servings—1 sandwich each

4 (3-ounce) minute steaks
1/3 cup fat-free Italian salad dressing
nonstick cooking spray
4 Italian rolls, sliced in half
1 ounce part-skim mozzarella cheese, shredded
1 cup fresh spinach, chopped

1. Prick steaks with a fork 6 times on each side. Marinate steaks in a shallow bowl with the Italian dressing for at least 15 minutes.

2. Spray a skillet with cooking spray, and heat over medium heat for 2 minutes. Add steaks, and cook for 4 minutes on each side.

3. Cut Italian rolls in half. Divide cheese and spinach among the 4 rolls. Place one steak on each roll, and serve.

255 calories per serving
7 gm. fat, 30 gm. protein, 18 gm. carbohydrate,
64 mg. cholesterol, 216 mg. sodium.

For exchange diets, count: 1 starch,
4 very lean meat, 1 vegetable.

Grilled Pork Chops with Fruit Salsa

Preparation time: 15 minutes
Marinating time: at least 30 minutes

4 servings—1 pork chop + 1/3 cup salsa each

Salsa:
>   16-ounce can chunky mixed fruit, drained
>   1 green onion, diced
>   2 tablespoons chopped fresh cilantro
>   2 tablespoons lemon juice
>   1/2 teaspoon minced garlic
>   1/4 teaspoon salt
>   1 jalapeño pepper, chopped fine

>   4 (3-ounce) pork chops, trimmed well

1. Combine ingredients for the salsa in a covered dish. Refrigerate for at least 30 minutes for the flavors to blend.

2. Grill trimmed pork chops over medium flame to desired doneness. Serve with fruit salsa on the side.

191 calories per serving
4 gm. fat, 25 gm. protein, 13 gm. carbohydrate,
65 mg. cholesterol, 385 mg. sodium.

For exchange diets, count: 1 fruit, 3 1/2 very lean meat.

Indian Chicken in the Crockpot

Preparation time: 20 minutes
Cooking time: 4-6 hours

8 servings—2 cups each

1 large onion, diced
4 boneless skinless chicken breast fillets, diced
2 carrots, washed and sliced into 1-inch chunks
2 red potatoes, washed and cut into chunks
14-ounce can chunky tomatoes
14-ounce can garbanzo beans, drained
1/4 cup golden raisins
1/2 teaspoon minced garlic
1/2 teaspoon ground ginger
1/2 teaspoon cumin
1/2 teaspoon turmeric
1/2 teaspoon black pepper
1/4 teaspoon salt
dash of cinnamon
dash of cayenne pepper
2 tablespoons dried parsley

1. Combine all ingredients in a Crockpot in the order listed. Use a long handled spoon to mix ingredients. Cook on high power for 4 to 6 hours. Serve as a stew in a soup bowl or over couscous.

204 calories per serving
2 gm. fat, 18 gm. protein, 29 gm. carbohydrate,
37 mg. cholesterol, 322 mg. sodium.

For exchange diets, count: 1 starch,
1 fruit, 2 very lean meat.

Lime and Ginger Shrimp Kabobs

Preparation time: 15 minutes
Marinating time: at least 30 minutes
Grilling time: 10 minutes

4 servings—4 to 5 ounces each

1 pound peeled deveined shrimp

Marinade:
    6 tablespoons lime juice
    3 tablespoons pineapple juice
    2 tablespoons rice wine vinegar
    1 tablespoon olive oil
    1/2 teaspoon dried coriander
    1 teaspoon ground ginger
    1/4 teaspoon red pepper flakes

    1 red pepper, seeded and cut into 1-inch pieces
    1 small red onion, quartered and separated into chunks
    1 firm kiwifruit, peeled and sliced into 8 coins

1. Place shrimp in a shallow container.

2. Combine ingredients for the marinade in a shaker container and blend well. Pour over the shrimp, cover and refrigerate for at least 30 minutes.

3. Thread marinated shrimp with pepper, onion, and kiwi on 4 skewers. Grill or broil, 4 minutes per side, turning skewers once, until shrimp are cooked through.

155 calories per serving
5 gm. fat, 25 gm. protein, 5 gm. carbohydrate,
173 mg. cholesterol, 168 mg. sodium.

For exchange diets, count: 1 vegetable, 4 lean meat.

Low-Fat Sausage Patties

Serve with low-fat pancakes or French toast.

Preparation time: 15 minutes
Cooking time: 15 minutes

8 servings—2 ounces each

1 pound lean pork
1/2 teaspoon salt
1/2 teaspoon black pepper
1/2 teaspoon paprika
1 teaspoon ground sage
1 tablespoon dried onion
1/4 cup beer or sugar-free cola
1/4 cup dry bread crumbs
nonstick cooking spray

1. Combine all ingredients in a mixing bowl, and form into 8 patties. Spray a nonstick skillet with cooking spray. Heat over medium heat. Brown patties for 7 to 8 minutes on each side, until pork is fully cooked.

109 calories per serving
3 gm. fat, 16 gm. protein, 3 gm. carbohydrate,
43 mg. cholesterol, 70 mg. sodium.

For exchange diets, count: 2 lean meat.

Muffin-Size Meatloaves

Preparation time: 15 minutes
Baking time: 30 minutes

8 servings—1 muffin meatloaf each

1 pound lean ground beef
1/4 cup dry vegetable soup mix
1 cup bread crumbs
1 teaspoon oregano
1/2 cup tomato juice or vegetable juice
nonstick cooking spray

1. Preheat oven to 400°.

2. Mix first five ingredients together in a mixing bowl.

3. Spray 8 muffin cups with cooking spray. Mound the meatloaf mixture up in the prepared cups, smoothing the tops. Bake for 30 minutes or until the center of the meatloaf is no longer pink.

166 calories per serving
6 gm. fat, 16 gm. protein, 11 gm. carbohydrate,
47 mg. cholesterol, 242 mg. sodium.

For exchange diets, count: 2 vegetable, 2 lean meat.

Nonfat Fried Chicken

Preparation time: 15 minutes
Baking time: 30 minutes

4 servings—4-5 ounces each

nonstick cooking spray
3 tablespoons grated Parmesan cheese
1/2 cup dry bread crumbs
1/2 teaspoon rosemary
1/2 teaspoon thyme
1/4 teaspoon garlic powder
1/4 teaspoon onion powder
1/4 teaspoon black pepper
4 chicken breast halves, skinned, deboned, and patted dry
3/4 cup low-fat buttermilk

1. Preheat oven to 400°.

2. Cover a baking sheet with aluminum foil and spray with cooking spray.

3. Combine all ingredients except chicken and buttermilk in a shallow dish. Pour buttermilk into another shallow dish. Dip chicken in the buttermilk, then roll in dry mixture, and set on baking sheet. Bake chicken for 25 to 30 minutes, until golden brown.

183 calories per serving
3 gm. fat, 32 gm. protein, 5 gm. carbohydrate,
45 mg. cholesterol, 313 mg. sodium.

For exchange diets, count: 5 very lean meat.

One-Dish Oven Beef Stew

Preparation time: 20 minutes
Baking time: 4 hours

8 servings—1 1/2 each

1 pound stew meat, trimmed well, and cut into 1-inch pieces
3 cups no-added-salt beef broth
2 large potatoes, peeled and cut into chunks
4 carrots, cleaned and cut into chunks
3 ribs of celery, diced
1 large onion, peeled and quartered
16-ounce can chunky tomatoes
1 teaspoon oregano
1/2 teaspoon thyme
1/2 teaspoon pepper
1 tablespoon Kitchen Bouquet browning sauce
1 teaspoon dried parsley

1. Combine all ingredients in a deep baking dish. Cover and bake at 325° for at least 4 hours. Stew may be baked as long as 6 hours. Remove cover during last 45 minutes of cooking.

182 calories per serving
5 gm. fat, 19 gm. protein, 15 gm. carbohydrate,
47 mg. cholesterol, 647 mg. sodium.

For exchange diets, count: 2 lean meat, 1 starch.

Orange 'n Spice Grilled Pork Chops

Preparation time: 30 minutes
Grilling time: 25 minutes

4 servings—3 ounce chop each

1 pound lean pork chops, scored in a crisscross pattern
1/4 cup frozen orange juice concentrate
1/4 teaspoon ground cloves
1 tablespoon Dijon mustard
garnish: orange slices

1. Trim pork well. Broil or grill until nearly done (7 to 10 minutes on each side).

2. Combine the next 3 ingredients and pour half of the mixture over chops. Broil or grill 2 more minutes. Turn chops, and pour remaining sauce on other side. Broil or grill 2 more minutes. Serve garnished with an orange slice.

225 calories per serving
9 gm. fat, 21 gm. protein, 11 gm. carbohydrate,
83 mg. cholesterol, 115 mg. sodium.

For exchange diets, count: 3 lean meat, 1 fruit.

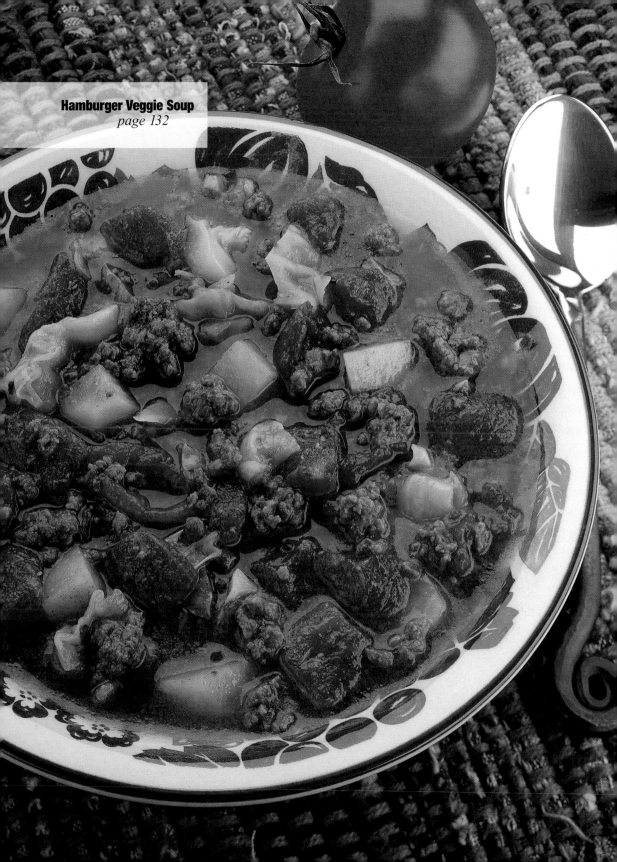

Hamburger Veggie Soup
page 132

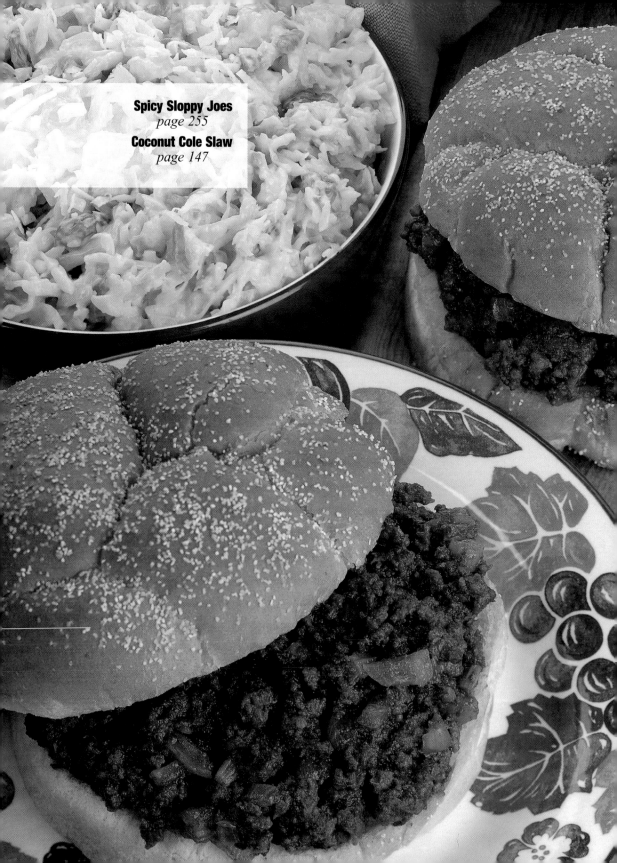

Spicy Sloppy Joes
page 255

Coconut Cole Slaw
page 147

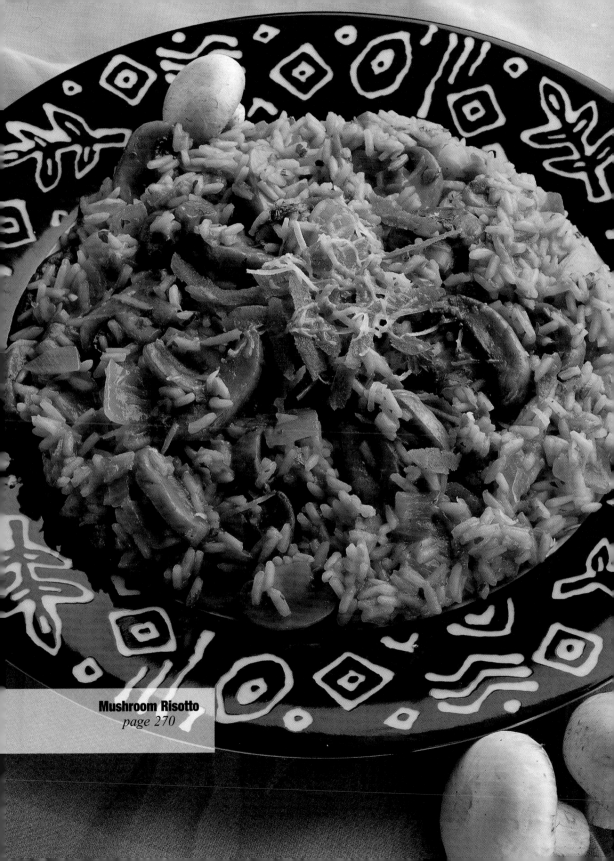

Mushroom Risotto
page 270

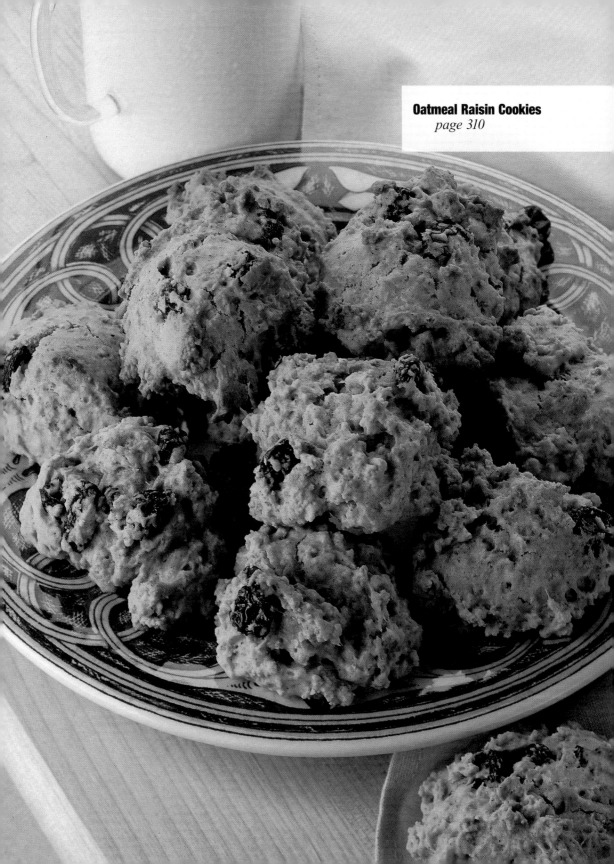

Oatmeal Raisin Cookies
page 310

Pepsi and Pork in the Crockpot

Thank you, Deb Preston.

Preparation time: 10 minutes
Cooking time: 4-6 hours
4 servings—3 ounces each

10-ounce can reduced-fat cream of mushroom soup
2 tablespoons reduced-sodium soy sauce
12 ounce Diet Pepsi
4 (3-ounce) pork chops, trimmed well (or substitute a pork roast)

1. Mix the soup, soy sauce, and Diet Pepsi together in the bottom of the Crockpot. Place the chops in the mixture, and slow cook on medium or high setting for 4 to 6 hours. Meat will be very tender.

213 calories per serving
9 gm. fat, 25 gm. protein, 6 gm. carbohydrate,
66 mg. cholesterol, 434 mg. sodium.

For exchange diets, count: 1/2 starch, 3 lean meat.

Poultry Marinade

Preparation time: 10 minutes
Marinating time: at least 30 minutes

8 servings—1 1/2 tablespoons each

2 tablespoons vegetable oil
1/4 cup lemon juice
1/2 teaspoon minced garlic
1 tablespoon chicken-flavor low-sodium bouillon powder
1/2 cup water
1/2 cup no-alcohol beer or white wine, or apple juice
1 1/2 teaspoons thyme

1. Combine all ingredients in a shaker container. Refrigerate for up to 3 months. Use with chicken and turkey breast fillets.

2. Marinate poultry in a shallow covered container in the refrigerator for at least 30 minutes. Always discard marinade after use. Use half the batch (about 3/4 cup) with 4 chicken breasts.

40 calories per serving
3 gm. fat, 0 protein, 0 carbohydrate,
0 cholesterol, 2 mg. sodium.

For exchange diets, count: 1 fat.

Roast Cornish Hen with Apple Stuffing

Preparation time: 20 minutes
Standing time: 15 minutes
Roasting time: 2 1/2 hours

4 servings—1/2 hen each

2 Cornish hens
1/2 teaspoon ground marjoram

Stuffing:
3 cups soft bread crumbs
1 tart apple, chopped
2 stalks celery with leaves, chopped
1 medium onion, chopped
1 tablespoon margarine, melted
1/2 teaspoon salt
1 teaspoon sage
1/2 teaspoon thyme
1/4 teaspoon pepper
1 cup apple juice

1. Trim excess fat from hens. Rub cavity of hens with marjoram. Fold wings across back with tips touching.

2. Stir ingredients for stuffing together in a medium-size bowl, then fill the body cavity lightly with stuffing.

3. Prick skin all over with a fork. Place hens, breast side up on rack in shallow roasting pan. Roast uncovered in 350° oven until done, about 2 1/2 hours, removing excess fat from the pan with a kitchen syringe. When meat is done, remove it to a platter, and allow to stand for 15 minutes for easier slicing.

446 calories per serving
9 gm. fat, 36 gm. protein, 53 gm. carbohydrate,
79 mg. cholesterol, 273 mg. sodium.

For exchange diets, count: 2 starch, 1 fruit,
1 vegetable, 3 1/2 lean meat.

Salmon Loaf

Preparation time: 15 minutes
Baking time: 30 minutes

4 servings—4 ounces each

nonstick cooking spray
1-pound can red or pink salmon, drained and flaked
8 soda crackers, crushed
1 egg, beaten or 1/4 cup liquid egg substitute
10-ounce can reduced-fat cream of celery soup
1 tablespoon lemon juice
1/4 teaspoon salt
1/4 teaspoon white pepper

1. Preheat oven to 400°. Spray a 1-quart baking dish with cooking spray.

2. Combine all ingredients in a medium mixing bowl.

3. Spread salmon mixture in the baking dish and bake for 30 minutes.

204 calories per serving
6 gm. fat, 26 gm. protein, 10 carbohydrate,
49 mg. cholesterol with egg substitute
(92 mg. cholesterol with egg), 1011 mg. sodium
(to reduce sodium, use unsalted crackers and fresh or frozen salmon).

For exchange diets, count: 1/2 starch, 3 lean meat.

Salmon Patties

Preparation time: 15 minutes
Cooking time: 16 minutes

4 servings—4 ounces each

nonstick cooking spray
1-pound can red or pink salmon, drained and flaked
8 soda crackers, crushed
1 egg, beaten, or 1/4 cup liquid egg substitute
1 tablespoon lemon juice
1/4 teaspoon salt
1/4 teaspoon white pepper

1. Spray a nonstick skillet with cooking spray. Heat over medium heat.

2. Combine all remaining ingredients in a medium mixing bowl. Form salmon mixture into 4 patties.

3. Cook patties over medium heat until brown (about 8 minutes). Turn and cook on the other side for about 8 minutes.

196 calories per serving
7 gm. fat, 25 gm. protein, 6 gm. carbohydrate,
49 mg. cholesterol with egg substitute
(92 mg. sodium with egg), 713 mg. sodium
(to reduce sodium, use unsalted crackers and fresh or frozen salmon).

For exchange diets, count: 1/2 starch, 3 lean meat.

Scallop Kabobs Basted with Garlic

Preparation time: 10 minutes
Grilling time: 15 minutes

4 servings—1 skewer each

2 large green peppers, cut into 1 1/2 inch squares
1 pound fresh scallops
1 pint cherry tomatoes

Sauce:
    1/4 cup dry white wine
    1 tablespoon vegetable oil
    2 tablespoons lemon juice
    1/2 teaspoon minced garlic
    1/2 teaspoon black pepper

1. Alternately thread first three ingredients on 4 skewers.

2. Combine ingredients for the sauce in a shaker container.

3. Grill kabobs for 15 minutes, turning several times and basting frequently with sauce.

179 calories per serving
5 gm. fat, 21 gm. protein, 12 gm. carbohydrate,
38 mg. cholesterol, 194 mg. sodium.

For exchange diets, count: 2 vegetables, 2 1/2 lean meat.

Seafood and Asparagus Stir-Fry

Preparation time: 15 minutes
Cooking time: 15 minutes

8 servings—1 1/2 cups each

1 pound salmon, orange roughy, shrimp, or scallops
1 tablespoon vegetable oil
10 ounces fresh or frozen asparagus
2 green onions, diced
2 ribs celery, sliced diagonally
4 ounces fresh mushrooms, washed, stemmed, and sliced
8-ounce can sliced water chestnuts, drained
2 cups chicken broth
2 tablespoons cornstarch
2 tablespoons reduced-sodium soy sauce

1. In a wok or large skillet, cook seafood in oil until it is white and flakes easily with a fork. Remove cooked fish from the pan and set aside. Add asparagus, onions, celery, and mushrooms to the pan. Stir-fry for 3 minutes or just until crisp. Add water chestnuts and chicken broth, and cook to boiling.

2. Combine cornstarch with soy sauce in a glass measuring cup or a small bowl, and add it to the hot mixture, stirring constantly. Continue cooking for 3 minutes until the mixture is thick. Toss in cooked seafood to heat through. Serve immediately over hot rice.

119 calories per serving
3 gm. fat, 14 gm. protein, 11 gm. carbohydrate,
15 mg. cholesterol, 332 mg. sodium.

For exchange diets, count: 2 vegetables, 1 lean meat.

Seafood Marinade

Preparation time: 10 minutes
Marinating time: at least 30 minutes

8 servings—1 1/2 tablespoons each

1/3 cup lemon juice
1/4 cup vegetable oil
1 teaspoon chicken-flavored low-sodium instant bouillon powder
1 teaspoon dill weed
1/3 cup dry white wine or rice vinegar or pineapple juice
1/2 cup water

1. Combine all ingredients in a shaker container. Refrigerate for up to 3 months. Use to perk up salmon, halibut, shrimp, or scallops before grilling or broiling.

2. Marinate seafood in a shallow covered container in the refrigerator for at least 30 minutes. Always discard marinade after use. Use half the batch (about 3/4 cup) with 4 fillets.

67 calories per serving
7 gm. fat, 0 protein, 0 carbohydrate,
0 cholesterol, 0 sodium.

For exchange diets, count: 1 1/2 fat.

Slow Cook Roast Pork with Braised Apples and Onions

Preparation time: 15 minutes
Cooking time: 4-6 hours

8 servings—4 ounces meat + 1/2 cup fruit and vegetable each

1 teaspoon minced garlic
1/2 teaspoon curry powder
1/4 teaspoon pepper
2 pounds boneless pork roast
4 large Golden Delicious apples, peeled and quartered
2 large onions, peeled and quartered
1 cup apple cider

1. Rub garlic, curry powder, and pepper over roast. Place in the Crockpot. Arrange apple and onion slices on top and around the pork. Pour apple cider over all. Cook on high heat for 4 to 6 hours.

252 calories per serving
6 gm. fat, 32 gm. protein, 17 gm. carbohydrate,
87 mg. cholesterol, 81 mg. sodium.

For exchange diets, count: 1 vegetable,
1 fruit, 4 1/2 very lean meat.

Spaghetti with Shrimp and Artichokes

Preparation time: 15 minutes
Cooking time: 10 minutes

4 servings—2 cups each

6 ounces spaghetti
16-ounce can seasoned crushed tomatoes with Italian herbs
8 ounces raw shrimp, peeled and deveined
1 cup sliced artichoke hearts, drained
garnish: 1 teaspoon dried basil

1. Prepare spaghetti according to package directions, taking care not to overcook it.

2. Meanwhile, combine shrimp, tomatoes, and artichoke hearts in a medium skillet. Cook over medium heat for 5 minutes, until shrimp are no longer pink and are curled up. Serve shrimp sauce over hot spaghetti, and garnish with dried basil.

154 calories per serving
2 gm. fat, 16 gm. protein, 21 gm. carbohydrate,
87 mg. cholesterol, 426 mg. sodium.

For exchange diets, count: 1 vegetable,
1 starch, 1 lean meat.

Spicy Sloppy Joes

Preparation time: 15 minutes
Cooking time: 25 minutes

8 servings—2/3 cup each

1 pound lean ground beef, cooked and drained well
2 ribs celery, chopped fine
1 large onion, chopped fine
6-ounce can tomato paste
1/4 cup frozen apple or grape juice concentrate
1 tablespoon lemon juice
1 tablespoon chili powder
2 teaspoons yellow mustard
1/2 teaspoon minced garlic

1. Combine drained ground beef with all other ingredients in a deep skillet. Bring mixture to a boil, then reduce heat to a simmer for 15 minutes. Serve on hamburger rolls.

146 calories per serving
6 gm. fat, 16 gm. protein, 7 gm. carbohydrate,
47 mg. cholesterol, 78 mg. sodium.

For exchange diets, count: 1/2 fruit, 2 lean meat.

Theresa's Turkey Bundles

This delightful dish was served by fellow registered dietitian, Theresa Eberhardt, to our Upper Iowa Dietitians group.

Preparation time: 20 minutes
Baking time: 25 minutes

4 servings—1 bundle each

4 ounces reduced-fat cream cheese
2 tablespoons skim milk
1 teaspoon dill weed
8 ounces cooked turkey, diced
1 rib celery, diced fine
1 small onion, diced fine
8-ounce tube reduced-fat crescent rolls
nonstick cooking spray
garnish: dill weed

1. Preheat oven to 350°.

2. In a mixing bowl, beat cream cheese, milk, and dill weed until smooth. Stir in turkey, celery, and onions.

3. Unroll crescent rolls into 4 rectangles. Place on a nonstick baking sheet and use your finger to smudge out the perforations between the rolls, mending the dough into 4 rectangles.

4. Divide turkey mixture between the rolls. Bring each corner to the center and pinch dough together, forming a pouch. Spray the tops with cooking spray, and sprinkle with dill weed.

5. Bake for 20 to 25 minutes or until golden brown. Serve hot.

303 calories per serving
9 gm. fat, 25 gm. protein, 31 gm. carbohydrate,
49 mg. cholesterol, 811 mg. sodium.

For exchange diets, count: 2 starch, 2 1/2 lean meat.

Thai Marinade

Preparation time: 10 minutes
Marinating time: at least 30 minutes

8 servings—1 1/2 tablespoons each

3 tablespoons lemon juice
2 tablespoons vegetable oil
2 tablespoons reduced-sodium soy sauce
1/2 teaspoon minced garlic
1 teaspoon beef-flavored low-sodium instant bouillon
1/2 teaspoon red pepper flakes

1. Combine all ingredients in a shaker container. Refrigerate for up to 3 months. Use with steak teriyaki, beef stir-fry, or lamb.

2. Marinate red meats in a shallow covered container in the refrigerator for at least 30 minutes. Always discard marinade after use. Use half the batch (about 3/4 cup) with 4 small steaks.

33 calories per serving
3 gm. fat, 0 protein, 0 carbohydrate,
0 cholesterol, 261 mg. sodium.

For exchange diets, count: 1 fat.

Three-Way Marinade for Chicken

Preparation time: 15 minutes

4 servings—1/4 cup each

1/2 cup lemon juice
1/4 cup frozen orange juice concentrate

Choose one of the following:
1/4 cup reduced-sodium soy sauce
1 tablespoon rosemary leaves, crushed, or
1 teaspoon tarragon leaves

1. Combine lemon juice and orange juice concentrate in a shallow dish. Add one of the flavor ingredients. Use as a marinade for chicken breasts.

With soy sauce
15 calories per serving
0 fat, 0 protein, 4 gm. carbohydrate,
0 cholesterol, 660 mg. sodium.
For exchange diets, count: as a free food.

With rosemary or tarragon
15 calories per serving
0 fat, 0 protein, 4 gm. carbohydrate,
0 cholesterol, 0 sodium.
For exchange diets, count: as a free food.

Wagon Wheel Beef Casserole

Preparation time: 20 minutes
Cooking time: 20 minutes

4 servings—1 1/2 cup each

4 ounces wagon wheel pasta
1/2 pound shredded leftover roast beef or 1/2 pound lean ground
    beef, browned and drained
1 medium onion, chopped fine
2 (14-ounce) cans chili-style chunky tomatoes
2 ounces reduced-fat cheddar cheese, shredded

1. Cook wagon wheel pasta according to package directions, and drain well.

2. Combine cooked beef with onion and tomatoes in a deep skillet. Cook over medium heat while pasta is cooking. When pasta is done, fold it into the tomato and beef mixture. Heat through. Sprinkle the top with shredded cheese. Continue cooking over low heat for 5 more minutes. Serve with corn bread muffins.

243 calories per serving
8 gm. fat, 22 gm. protein, 24 gm. carbohydrate,
64 mg. cholesterol, 573 mg. sodium.

For exchange diets, count: 1 starch, 2 vegetable, 2 lean meat.

Chapter Eight

Vegetables
and
Side Dishes

Asparagus Almond Casserole

Preparation time: 10 minutes
Baking time: 20 minutes

8 servings—3/4 cup each

1-pound bag frozen asparagus spears, thawed
1/4 cup toasted almonds
1 can reduced-fat cream of chicken soup
1/2 cup cracked pepper cracker crumbs

1. Preheat oven to 375°.

2. Layer asparagus spears, almonds, and soup in a baking dish. Sprinkle with cracker crumbs, and bake for 20 minutes.

119 calories per serving
5 gm. fat, 5 gm. protein, 17 gm. carbohydrate,
1 mg. cholesterol, 240 mg. sodium.

For exchange diets, count: 1 vegetable, 1 fat, 1/2 skim milk.

Baked Bermuda Onions

Preparation time: 15 minutes
Baking time: 30 minutes

8 servings—3/4 cup each

nonstick cooking spray
2 pounds Bermuda onions, peeled and sliced thin
2 tablespoons flour
1 egg or 1/4 cup liquid egg substitute
1/2 teaspoon black pepper
1 tablespoon Worcestershire sauce
1 teaspoon hot pepper sauce
3/4 cup nonfat sour cream
3 ounces reduced-fat Swiss cheese, shredded

1. Preheat oven to 400°.

2. Spray an 11" x 7" casserole dish with cooking spray. Place onion slices in the prepared dish.

3. In a small mixing bowl, mix flour with egg until smooth. Add all remaining ingredients, and pour over the onion slices. Bake for 30 minutes or until the top of the casserole is golden brown.

99 calories per serving
1 gm. fat, 6 gm. protein, 17 gm. carbohydrate,
6 mg. cholesterol, 215 mg. sodium.

For exchange diets, count: 1 starch, 1 vegetable.

Barbecued Baked Beans

Preparation time: 10 minutes
Cooking time: 25 minutes

8 servings—1/2 cup each

2 slices bacon
1 small onion, diced
1/2 cup spicy ketchup
2 tablespoons vinegar
2 tablespoons water
1 teaspoon prepared mustard
1 teaspoon Worcestershire sauce
1/8 teaspoon salt
1/8 teaspoon black pepper
24-ounce can Great Northern beans, drained
1/4 cup Nutrasweet Spoonful sugar substitute

1. In a deep skillet, cook bacon with onion until bacon is crisp. Spoon drippings from the pan, and then drain bacon and onion between two paper towels. Return onion and bacon to the skillet, and add all remaining ingredients except the sugar substitute. Cook over medium heat for 15 minutes, then stir in sugar substitute and serve.

113 calories per serving
2 gm. fat, 7 gm. protein, 19 gm. carbohydrate,
2 mg. cholesterol, 239 mg. sodium.

For exchange diets, count: 1 1/2 starch.

Brussels Sprouts with Mustard Sauce

Preparation time: 15 minutes
Cooking time: 8 minutes

8 servings—3/4 cup each

1 pound fresh brussels sprouts, cleaned and trimmed
2 tablespoons soft margarine
1 1/2 tablespoons lemon juice
1 teaspoon finely grated lemon peel
1 1/2 teaspoons mustard seeds
1/4 teaspoon salt
1/4 teaspoon pepper

1. Use a knife to carve a small "X" in the stem end of the sprouts. Place sprouts in a microwave-safe dish. Sprinkle with 2 tablespoons of water, cover, and cook on high power for 6 minutes.

2. In a small skillet, melt margarine. Stir in all remaining ingredients. Cook and stir over low heat. When sprouts are done, drain well and toss in the skillet, stirring to coat the vegetables with the sauce. Serve hot.

34 calories per serving
2 gm. fat, 2 gm. protein, 5 gm. carbohydrate,
0 cholesterol, 45 mg. sodium.

For exchange diets, count: 1 vegetable.

Broccoli with Orange Sauce

Preparation time: 15 minutes
Cooking time: 6 minutes

8 servings—3/4 cup each

1 large bunch fresh broccoli
1/2 cup no-added-salt chicken broth
1/2 cup orange juice
1 teaspoon cornstarch
1 green onion, sliced thin
1/2 teaspoon dried basil
1/4 teaspoon salt
1/4 teaspoon pepper
1 seeded orange, peeled and chopped

1. Wash, trim and chop broccoli. Place in a microwave-safe dish, sprinkle with 1 tablespoon of water, cover and cook on high power for 6 minutes.

2. Meanwhile, in a small saucepan, combine broth and orange juice with cornstarch. Cook over medium heat, stirring constantly until thickened. Stir in all remaining ingredients.

3. Transfer steamed broccoli to a serving bowl. Toss with orange sauce, and serve.

28 calories per serving
0 fat, 1 gm. protein, 6 gm. carbohydrate,
0 cholesterol, 78 mg. sodium.

For exchange diets, count: 1 vegetable.

Buttermilk Onion and Garlic Mashed Potatoes

Preparation time: 5 minutes
Cooking time: 7 minutes

4 servings—3/4 cup each

1/2 cup low-fat buttermilk
1 cup milk
1 1/2 cups instant mashed potato flakes
1/2 teaspoon minced garlic
1/2 teaspoon onion powder
1/2 teaspoon white pepper

1. In a microwave-safe bowl, cook buttermilk and milk 5 minutes on high power or until bubbles appear around the outside of the bowl. Whisk in all remaining ingredients. Cook 2 more minutes on high power, and serve.

129 calories per serving
5 gm. fat, 5 gm. protein, 17 gm. carbohydrate,
14 mg. cholesterol, 346 mg. sodium.

For exchange diets, count: 1 starch, 1 fat.

Cranberry Compote for Turkey or Pork

Preparation time: 5 minutes
Cooking time: 11 minutes

16 servings—1/4 cup each

1 teaspoon vegetable oil
1 medium onion, finely chopped
8 ounces fresh cranberries
1/2 teaspoon allspice
1/2 teaspoon cinnamon
12-ounce jar all-fruit orange marmalade
8-ounce can crushed pineapple in juice, drained well

1. Heat oil in a medium saucepan. Add onion, and cook for 3 minutes or until soft. Add all remaining ingredients, and cook uncovered over medium heat for 8 minutes. Serve this compote warm or cold with roast turkey or pork.

84 calories per serving
0 fat, 0 protein, 21 gm. carbohydrate,
0 cholesterol, 32 mg. sodium.

For exchange diets, count: 1 1/2 fruit.

Green Beans with a Bite

Preparation time: 5 minutes
Cooking time: 20 minutes

4 servings—1 cup each

1 teaspoon olive oil
1 medium onion, chopped fine
1/2 teaspoon minced garlic
16-ounce can chopped tomatoes
1 teaspoon finely grated lemon rind
1 teaspoon hot pepper sauce
sugar substitute equivalent to 1/2 teaspoon sugar
16-ounce can French-style green beans, drained well

1. Heat olive oil in a skillet. Add onion and garlic, and cook for 4 minutes or until onion is soft. Add all remaining ingredients, and continue cooking uncovered over medium heat for 15 minutes. Juice from tomatoes should be evaporated away.

73 calories per serving
2 gm. fat, 3 gm. protein, 15 gm. carbohydrate,
0 cholesterol, 568 mg. sodium
(to reduce sodium, choose no-added-salt green beans).

For exchange diets, count: 3 vegetable.

Mushroom Risotto

Preparation time: 10 minutes
Cooking time: 25 minutes

8 servings—3/4 cup each

3 cups no-added-salt vegetable broth
1 teaspoon olive oil
1 large yellow onion, diced
1/4 teaspoon minced garlic
8 ounces fresh mushrooms, cleaned, stemmed and sliced
1 large carrot, washed and grated
1 cup short grain rice
1/4 cup freshly grated Parmesan cheese
1/4 cup chopped fresh Italian parsley

1. In a medium saucepan, heat broth over high heat to boiling.

2. Heat oil in a large skillet over medium heat, then add onion and garlic, cooking for 4 minutes or until the onion is soft. Stir in mushrooms and carrots, and continue cooking for 5 more minutes. Add rice to the vegetable mixture in the skillet. Then add the boiling vegetable broth, 1/2 to 3/4 cup at a time, stirring constantly until all the broth has been added. Continue cooking over low heat for 15 minutes. Stir in cheese and parsley, and serve.

70 calories per serving
2 gm. fat, 3 gm. protein, 11 gm. carbohydrate,
2 mg. cholesterol, 73 mg. sodium.

For exchange diets, count: 1/2 starch, 1 vegetable.

Old-Fashioned Fried Potatoes

Preparation time: 10 minutes
Cooking time: 15 minutes

4 servings—3/4 cup each

4 small or 2 large potatoes, washed, peeled, and sliced
2 tablespoons water
2 teaspoons vegetable oil
1/2 teaspoon salt
1/4 teaspoon pepper

1. Place potato slices in a microwave-safe dish, and sprinkle with water. Cover and cook on high power for 8 minutes. Remove cover.

2. Heat oil in a large nonstick skillet over medium heat. Spoon steamed potato slices into the skillet. Brown the potatoes over medium heat for 5 to 7 minutes. Season with salt and pepper, and serve.

78 calories per serving
2 gm. fat, 1 gm. protein, 14 gm. carbohydrate,
0 cholesterol, 141 mg. sodium.

For exchange diets, count: 1 starch.

Potato Casserole in the Microwave

Preparation time: 10 minutes
Cooking time: 15 minutes

8 servings—3/4 cup each

nonstick cooking spray
16-ounce can sliced potatoes, drained
16-ounce can whole kernel corn, drained
14-ounce can chopped green chilies, drained
1/4 teaspoon black pepper
1/2 cup low-fat buttermilk
1 tablespoon flour
2 ounces reduced-fat Monterey jack cheese, shredded

1. Spray an 11" x 7" casserole dish with cooking spray. Mix the potatoes, corn, and chilies together in the dish. Sprinkle with black pepper.

2. In a glass measure, whisk flour and buttermilk together. Then pour over the potato mixture, and cover. Microwave for 10 minutes on 70% power. Sprinkle cheese over the top and cook at 70% for 5 more minutes.

125 calories per serving
3 gm. fat, 5 gm. protein, 22 gm. carbohydrate,
0 cholesterol, 731 mg. sodium
(*to reduce sodium, choose no-added-salt corn and potatoes*).

For exchange diets, count: 1 1/2 starch.

Rice with Nuts and Spice

Preparation time: 10 minutes
Cooking time: 8 minutes

4 servings—3/4 cup each

1 cup instant rice
1 cup no-added-salt chicken broth
1 teaspoon margarine
1 small onion, finely chopped
1 large carrot, cleaned and shredded
2 tablespoons chopped walnuts
1/2 teaspoon marjoram
1/2 teaspoon thyme
1/2 teaspoon rosemary
4-ounce can sliced mushrooms, drained
2 tablespoons chopped parsley

1. Place rice and broth in a microwave-safe dish. Cover with plastic wrap, and cook on high for 3 minutes.

2. Meanwhile, combine all remaining ingredients in a skillet, and cook over medium heat until onions and carrot are soft. Stir vegetables, nuts, and spices into the hot rice, and serve.

119 calories per serving
5 gm. fat, 4 gm. protein, 54 gm. carbohydrate,
0 cholesterol, 37 mg. sodium.

For exchange diets, count: 1 starch, 1 fat.

Scalloped Corn

Preparation time: 15 minutes
Baking time: 30 minutes

4 servings—3/4 cup each

nonstick cooking spray
1-pound can fat-free cream-style corn
2 eggs or 1/2 cup liquid egg substitute
1 cup skim milk
1/4 teaspoon salt
1/2 teaspoon white pepper
dash of nutmeg
8 soda crackers, crushed fine
garnish: dried parsley

1. Preheat oven to 400°.

2. Spray a medium casserole dish with cooking spray. Combine all ingredients in the casserole dish, stirring to blend. Sprinkle dried parsley on the top. Bake for 30 minutes or until mixture is set.

155 calories per serving
2 gm. fat, 8 gm. protein, 30 gm. carbohydrate,
2 mg. cholesterol with egg substitute
(86 mg. cholesterol with egg), 468 mg. sodium.

For exchange diets, count: 2 starch.

Summer Fruit on the Grill

Preparation time: 15 minutes

4 servings—1 kabob each

3 plums, halved
4 apricots, halved
2 peaches, cut into 4 wedges
2 pears, cut into 4 wedges
2 bananas, cut into 4 chunks
1/2 cup pineapple chunks
2 tablespoons lemon juice
1/4 teaspoon cinnamon

Dressing:
2 cups nonfat sugar-free plain yogurt
1 teaspoon vanilla
sugar substitute equivalent to 1/4 cup sugar

1. Pit or core fruit. Leave peelings on the fruit. Place in a shallow pan or dish and sprinkle with lemon juice. Thread pieces of fruit on 4 skewers. Each skewer will have 2 pieces of each fruit. Sprinkle with cinnamon.

2. Place on grill over medium flame for 2 minutes. Turn kabobs once. Grill 2 minutes more on opposite side.

3. Meanwhile, combine dressing ingredients. Remove kabobs from grill, and transfer to single dessert dishes. Top with dressing and serve.

220 calories per serving
0 fat, 4 gm. protein, 50 gm. carbohydrate,
0 cholesterol, 49 mg. sodium.

For exchange diets, count: 3 fruit,78

Summer Peas with Bacon

Preparation time: 10 minutes
Cooking time: 15 minutes

8 servings—1/2 cup each

1 pound package frozen baby peas
3 slices bacon, diced
2 green onions, chopped fine
1/4 cup herb vinegar
1 teaspoon flour
sugar substitute equivalent to 2 tablespoons sugar (recipe tested
    with Equal Measure)

1. Place peas in a microwave-safe dish, cover with plastic wrap, and microwave for 4 to 6 minutes.

2. Meanwhile, cook bacon and onion in a medium skillet over medium-high heat until the bacon is crisp. Remove bacon and onion to a paper towel, and discard drippings from the pan.

3. Pour vinegar in the skillet. Whisk flour into the vinegar. Cook over medium heat, stirring constantly until thick. Stir sugar substitute, bacon, and onion into the mixture and pour sauce over the peas, and serve.

64 calories per serving
1 gm. fat, 4 gm. protein, 10 gm. carbohydrate,
2 mg. cholesterol, 88 mg. sodium.

For exchange diets, count: 2 vegetables.

Summer Veggies on the Grill

Preparation time: 15 minutes
Marinating time: 20 minutes
Grilling time: 12 minutes

8 servings—3/4 cup each

Marinade:
  1/2 cup chopped parsley
  1/4 cup red wine vinegar
  2 teaspoons chopped onion
  1/4 teaspoon garlic powder
  1 teaspoon Worcestershire sauce
  1/4 teaspoon pepper
  1 tablespoon vegetable oil

  1 eggplant, peeled and cut into 1/2-inch-thick rounds
  2 zucchini, cut into 1-inch chunks

1. Combine ingredients for marinade in a shaker container. Place eggplant, zucchini, and marinade in a heavy zippered plastic bag. Marinate for 15 minutes.

2. Grill on aluminum foil or on a kabob stick over medium coals, turning once, until tender, 10 to 12 minutes.

95 calories per serving
4 gm. fat, 4 gm. protein, 10 gm. carbohydrate,
0 cholesterol, 62 mg. sodium.

For exchange diets, count: 2 vegetable, 1 fat.

Sweet and Tangy Microwave Carrots

Preparation time: 10 minutes
Cooking time: 6 minutes

4 servings—3/4 cup each

1 pound fresh carrots
2 tablespoons lemon juice
2 tablespoons firmly-packed brown sugar
   or Sugar Twin brown sugar substitute
1/3 cup raisins
1 tablespoon soft margarine

1. Choose firm, clean, well-shaped carrots with bright orange-gold color. Scrub clean, peel, and slice carrots into coins. Place in a 2-quart microwave-safe dish. Sprinkle with lemon juice, brown sugar, and raisins. Cover. Microwave on high power for 6 minutes. Carrots will be tender-crisp. For softer carrots, increase cooking time by 1 minute. Dot with margarine and serve.

132 calories per serving
(105 calories with sugar substitute)
0 fat, 2 gm. protein, 30 gm. carbohydrate
(23 gm. carbohydrate with sugar substitute),
0 cholesterol, 71 mg. sodium.

For exchange diets, count: 1 vegetable,
1 1/2 fruit, 1/2 fat.
(Count 1 vegetable, 1 fruit, 1/2 fat with sugar substitute.)

Sweet Potato Revenge

Preparation time: 15 minutes
Baking time: 30 minutes

8 servings—3/4 cup each

nonstick cooking spray
2 (16-ounce) cans sweet potatoes or yams, drained, and then mashed
1/2 cup orange juice concentrate
1/2 cup skim milk
1 teaspoon vanilla
1 teaspoon cinnamon
2 tablespoons chopped pecans

1. Preheat oven to 375°.

2. Spray an 11" x 7" baking dish with cooking spray.

3. In a mixing bowl, combine all ingredients except the pecans. Spread sweet potato mixture in the prepared casserole dish. Sprinkle pecans on top, and bake for 30 minutes.

169 calories per serving
3 gm. fat, 3 gm. protein, 35 gm. carbohydrate,
0 cholesterol, 18 mg. sodium.

For exchange diets, count: 2 starch.

Twice-Baked Potatoes

Preparation time: 20 minutes
Baking time: 1 hour

8 servings—1 stuffed shell each

4 medium baking potatoes
1/2 cup nonfat sour cream
1 tablespoon reduced-fat margarine
1 teaspoon dill weed
1/2 teaspoon seasoned salt
1 tablespoon grated Parmesan cheese
4 drops hot pepper sauce

1. Preheat oven to 450°.

2. Wash potatoes well and place in the oven; bake for 50 minutes.

3. Using an oven mitt, remove potatoes from the oven and slice in half. Carefully scoop out the potato, leaving about 1/2 inch of pulp inside the shell. Remove pulp to a large bowl.

4. Mix pulp with all remaining ingredients and then stuff mixture back into the 8 shells. Return to the oven for 10 minutes.

82 calories per serving
1 gm. fat, 2 gm. protein, 17 gm. carbohydrate,
0 cholesterol, 51 mg. sodium.

For exchange diets, count: 1 starch.

Vegetable Relish for Broiled Fish

Preparation time: 15 minutes
Chilling time: 1 hour

4 servings—3/4 cup each

1 cup shredded carrots
1 cup chopped cucumber
1/2 cup chopped red pepper
1/4 cup finely chopped red onion
3 tablespoons cider vinegar
1 teaspoon Equal Measure sugar substitute
1/4 teaspoon salt
1 tablespoon vegetable oil

1. Combine carrot, cucumber, pepper, and onion in a medium bowl. Set aside.

2. Stir together vinegar, sugar substitute, and salt. Whisk in oil. Pour over vegetables, and toss to coat. Cover and refrigerate at least 1 hour before serving. Use as an accompaniment with ordinary broiled whitefish.

84 calories per serving
4 gm. fat, 4 gm. protein, 10 gm. carbohydrate,
0 cholesterol, 162 mg. sodium.

For exchange diets, count: 2 vegetable, 1 fat.

Wild Rice with Apricots

Preparation time: 10 minutes
Cooking time: 25 minutes

8 servings—3/4 cup each

6-ounce package brown rice and wild rice mix
1/3 cup no-added-salt chicken broth
1 small onion, cut into strips
16-ounce can apricot halves, drained and chopped
1/2 teaspoon sage
1/8 teaspoon pepper

1. Prepare rice mix according to package directions.

2. In a skillet, heat chicken broth and onion until onion is soft. Stir in diced apricots, sage, and pepper; heat through. When rice is done, pour apricot mixture over the rice, toss to mix, and transfer to a serving dish.

65 calories per serving
0 fat, 1 gm. protein, 15 gm. carbohydrate,
0 cholesterol, 5 mg. sodium.

For exchange diets, count: 1 fruit.

Chapter Nine

Desserts

Almond Custard

Preparation time: 15 minutes
Chilling time: 4 hours

4 servings—1/2 cup custard and 1/2 cup fruit each

3/4 cup water
1/4 cup sugar, or sugar substitute
1 envelope unflavored gelatin
1 cup skim milk
1 teaspoon almond extract
2 cups unsweetened fruit of choice

1. Heat water, sugar or substitute, and gelatin to boiling; stir until gelatin is dissolved. Remove from heat and stir in milk and almond extract.

2. Pour into a loaf dish. Cover and refrigerate until firm, at least 4 hours. Cut gelatin custard into 1-inch diamonds or squares. Place fruit in a serving bowl, and place the bowl on a platter. Arrange custard on the platter around the fruit. Serve custard with fruit on the side.

105 calories per serving
0 fat, 4 gm. protein, 13 gm. carbohydrate,
0 cholesterol, 82 mg. sodium.

For exchange diets, count: 1 fruit, 1/2 skim milk.

Apple Crunch

Preparation time: 20 minutes
Baking time: 30 minutes

8 servings—1/8 pan each

1 cup quick oats
3 tablespoons brown sugar,
   or 3 tablespoons Sugar Twin brown sugar substitute
2 tablespoons margarine, melted
1/2 teaspoon cinnamon
6 medium baking apples, peeled and sliced thin
1/4 cup water
1/4 cup brown sugar,
   or 1/4 cup Sugar Twin brown sugar substitute
2 tablespoons flour
1/2 teaspoon cinnamon

1. Preheat oven to 350°.

2 Combine oats, 3 tablespoons brown sugar or substitute, margarine, and cinnamon in a small mixing bowl; mix well.

3. In an 8" square baking dish, mix sliced apples and water with 1/4 cup brown sugar or substitute, flour, and cinnamon. Top with reserved oat mixture, and bake for 30 minutes.

139 calories per serving (93 calories without sugar)
2 gm. fat, 1 gm. protein, 31 gm. carbohydrate (19 gm. carbohydrate without sugar), 0 cholesterol, 30 mg. sodium.

For exchange diets, count: 1 starch, 1 fruit
(Count 1 fruit, 1/2 starch with sugar substitute).

Apple Pie with Crunch Topping

Preparation time: 20 minutes
Baking time: 45 minutes
Cooling time: 1 hour

10 servings—1 slice each

9-inch frozen single pie crust (such as Pet Ritz)
10 Golden Delicious apples, peeled and sliced very thin
2 tablespoons cornstarch
1 teaspoon cinnamon
1/2 cup frozen apple juice concentrate

Topping:
2 tablespoons soft margarine
1/3 cup oatmeal
1 teaspoon cinnamon
1/4 cup flour

1. Preheat oven to 350°.

2. Prick the pie crust with a fork 8 times.

3. Slice peeled apples into the crust. Sprinkle with cornstarch and cinnamon, and toss to coat. Pour apple juice concentrate over the apples.

4. In a small mixing bowl, combine ingredients for topping, stirring until crumbly. Spread over the top of the apples, and bake for 45 minutes. Cool 1 hour before slicing.

196 calories per serving
4 gm. fat, 2 gm. protein, 39 gm. carbohydrate,
0 cholesterol, 164 mg. sodium.

For exchange diets, count: 2 starch, 1/2 fruit.

Baked Apples with Raisin Sauce

Preparation time: 20 minutes
Baking time: 30 minutes

4 servings—1 apple each

4 large baking apples
2 tablespoons Sugar Twin brown sugar substitute, divided
1/2 teaspoon ground allspice, divided
2 teaspoons soft margarine, divided
1/4 cup golden raisins
2 tablespoons Sugar Twin Spoonable sweetener
1 1/2 teaspoons cornstarch
1 teaspoon finely grated orange peel
1/2 teaspoon cinnamon
1/8 teaspoon salt
1 1/2 cups boiling water
1 1/2 teaspoons rum or maple extract

1. Preheat oven to 375°.

2. Core apples and peel upper half of each apple.

3. Place apples in an 8" square baking dish. Season the center of each apple with Brown Sugar Twin, allspice, and margarine.

4. In a small bowl, combine raisins, Sugar Twin Spoonable, cornstarch, orange peel, cinnamon, and salt. Stir in boiling water and rum or maple extract with a whisk. Pour sauce over the prepared apples and bake for 30 minutes. Baste the apples several times with sauce.

151 calories per serving
2 gm. fat, 1 gm. protein, 40 gm. carbohydrate,
0 cholesterol, 114 mg. sodium.

For exchange diets, count: 2 fruit, 1/2 fat.

Banana Cream Pie

Preparation time: 20 minutes
Chilling time: 2 hours

8 servings—1 slice each

prepared reduced-fat graham cracker crust
2 firm ripe bananas
2 (3-ounce) packages sugar-free vanilla pudding
3 cups fat-free eggnog, or 3 cups skim milk
2 drops yellow food coloring
garnish: 8 whole fresh strawberries

1. Peel and slice bananas into the prepared crust.

2. Prepare pudding mix according to package directions using eggnog or skim milk. Stir yellow food coloring into the pudding; pour pudding over the bananas. Refrigerate at least 2 hours or until ready to serve. Garnish each portion with a fresh strawberry.

170 calories per serving
3 gm. fat, 5 gm. protein, 29 gm. carbohydrate,
2 mg. cholesterol, 229 mg. sodium.

For exchange diets, count: 1/2 skim milk, 1/2 fruit.

Banana Pudding

Preparation time: 10 minutes
Chilling time: 1 hour

8 servings—1/2 cup each

2 very ripe large bananas
2 cups sugar-free banana-flavored yogurt
1 cup reduced-fat sour cream
1/4 teaspoon nutmeg
1 teaspoon vanilla

1. Peel bananas and slice into a blender container. Add yogurt, and process on low power just until bananas are mashed smooth. Fold in sour cream, nutmeg, and vanilla, and pour into 8 dessert cups. Chill at least 1 hour or until serving time.

89 calories per serving
0 fat, 6 gm. protein, 17 gm. carbohydrate,
1 mg. cholesterol, 84 mg. sodium.

For exchange diets, count: 1 skim milk.

Cappuccino Parfait

Preparation time: 20 minutes

6 servings—2/3 cup each

3-ounce package sugar-free vanilla pudding
1 1/2 cups skim milk
2 teaspoons instant coffee granules
1 cup reduced-fat whipped topping
3 chocolate sandwich cookies
2 tablespoons sliced almonds

1. In a medium saucepan, combine pudding mix with milk and coffee granules. Prepare pudding according to package directions. Cool mixture to room temperature, then fold in whipped topping.

2. In a zippered plastic bag, crush sandwich cookies, and then mix with almonds.

3. Layer into 6 parfait glasses: pudding, sprinkle of cookies and almonds, pudding, and sprinkles of cookies and almonds. Refrigerate until ready to serve.

184 calories per serving
10 gm. fat, 4 gm. protein, 22 gm. carbohydrate,
1 mg. cholesterol, 70 mg. sodium.

For exchange diets, count: 1 1/2 fat, 1 1/2 starch.

Cheesecake with Strawberry Topping

Preparation time: 20 minutes
Baking time: 10 minutes
Chilling time: 3 hours

8 servings—1 slice each

Crust:
   2 cups graham crackers
   1 tablespoon melted margarine

Cheesecake filling:
   2 (3-ounce) packages sugar-free lemon gelatin
   3/4 cup boiling water
   2 tablespoons lemon juice
   2 cups low-fat cottage cheese
   1 cup evaporated skim milk
   2 cups sliced fresh strawberries

1. Preheat oven to 400°. Place a small mixing bowl in the refrigerator.

2. Combine graham cracker crumbs and margarine in a 9" pie dish or an 11" x 7" baking dish; pat to cover the bottom and sides. Bake for 10 minutes, until crumbs are lightly browned. Cool.

3. In a blender container, combine gelatin with boiling water. Blend on high until gelatin is dissolved. Add lemon juice and blend again. Add 1 cup of the cottage cheese to blender container. Blend the mixture until absolutely smooth, then add second cup. Transfer the mixture to a mixing bowl.

4. Whip the chilled evaporated skim milk in the chilled bowl until thick, and then fold into the cottage cheese mixture. Pour onto crust, and chill for 3 hours. Slice and serve with fresh berries on top.

215 calories per serving
6 gm. fat, 4 gm. protein, 22 gm. carbohydrate,
6 mg. cholesterol, 424 mg. sodium.

For exchange diets, count: 1 fruit, 1 fat, 1 1/2 skim milk.

Chewy Double Chocolate Cookies

Preparation time: 20 minutes
Baking time: 12 minutes

36 servings—1 cookie each

nonstick cooking spray
1/3 cup margarine
1/3 cup sugar, or 1/3 cup Sugar Twin Spoonable sweetener
1/3 cup brown sugar, or 1/3 cup Sugar Twin brown sugar substitute
1 egg
1/2 cup skim milk
2 teaspoons vanilla
2 cups quick oats
1 cup flour
1/3 cup cocoa
1 1/2 teaspoons baking powder
1/2 cup reduced-fat chocolate chips

1. Preheat oven to 350°.

2. Spray a baking sheet with cooking spray.

3. In a mixing bowl, beat margarine, sugars, and egg until creamy. Beat in milk and vanilla. Fold in oats, flour, cocoa, and baking powder.

4. Drop cookie dough by rounded tablespoons onto baking sheet. Bake for 6 minutes, then sprinkle tops with chocolate chips, and bake 6 more minutes. Cool for 1 minute before removing to a wire rack.

70 calories per serving (55 calories without sugar)
2 gm. fat, 1 gm. protein, 12 gm. carbohydrate (8 gm. carbohydrate with sugar substitute), 6 mg. cholesterol, 23 mg. sodium.

For exchange diets, count: 1 starch with sugar
(count 1/2 fruit, 1/2 fat with sugar substitute).

Chilled Raspberry Soup

Preparation time: 10 minutes
Chilling time: 30 minutes

4 servings—1 cup each

1 1/2 cups apple juice
1/2 cup evaporated skim milk
1 cup nonfat sour cream
2 teaspoons sugar-free raspberry drink powder (such as Kool-aid)
2 cups fresh raspberries, washed and sorted

1. In a large bowl, use a whisk to combine apple juice with skim milk; whisk the sour cream into the juice and milk. Stir in drink powder until fully dissolved. Fold in raspberries. Chill for at least 30 minutes. Serve.

93 calories per serving
0 fat, 1 gm. protein, 22 gm. carbohydrate,
0 cholesterol, 21 mg. sodium.

For exchange diets, count: 1 1/2 fruit.

Chocolate Almond Mousse

Preparation time: 20 minutes
Chilling time: 2 hours

8 servings—1/3 cup each

8-ounce package reduced-fat cream cheese
1/3 cup Equal Measure sugar substitute
1/4 cup cocoa
1 teaspoon vanilla extract
1 teaspoon almond extract
1 envelope unflavored gelatin
1/4 cup cold water
1/2 cup reduced-fat semisweet baking chips
1/2 cup skim milk
garnish: whole almonds

1. In a medium mixing bowl, combine softened cream cheese, sugar substitute, cocoa, and vanilla and almond extracts. Beat smooth.

2. In another small bowl, sprinkle gelatin over the water, and let stand 3 minutes to soften.

3. Place the chips and milk in a glass measuring cup, and microwave on high power for 1 to 1 1/2 minutes until chips are softened.

4. Add dissolved gelatin mixture and melted chocolate mixture slowly to the cream cheese mixture, beating with electric mixer on medium-low power. Transfer to dessert dishes, and refrigerate at least 2 hours or until serving time. Garnish each dish with several whole almonds.

99 calories per serving
4 gm. fat, 6 gm. protein, 13 gm. carbohydrate,
1 mg. cholesterol, 172 mg. sodium.

For exchange diets, count: 1 skim milk.

Chocolate Strawberries

Preparation time: 15 minutes

8 servings—1/2 cup each

1 quart fresh strawberries, washed
2 ounces (1/3 cup) reduced-fat semisweet baking chips

1. Prepare berries for dipping by washing well, and allowing to dry. Do not remove stems.

2. Place chips in a 1-cup glass measuring cup. Microwave on high power for 10 seconds, stir, cook on high for 10 more seconds, stir, then cook on high for 10 more seconds. Chips should be melted.

3. Use the stem or a fork to dip ends of berries into melted chocolate. Dry berries upside down on waxed paper. When dry, arrange on a platter, and serve.

48 calories per serving
2 gm. fat, 0 protein, 9 gm. carbohydrate,
0 cholesterol, 2 mg. sodium.

For exchange diets, count: 1/2 fruit, 1/2 fat.

Cran Apple Crisp

Preparation time: 20 minutes
Baking time: 40 minutes

12 servings—1/12 pan each

nonstick cooking spray
1/2 cup apple juice concentrate
3 tablespoons flour
1 teaspoon finely grated orange peel
6 large baking apples, peeled and sliced thin
1 cup whole cranberries

Topping:
2 cups low-fat granola

1. Preheat oven to 375°.

2. Spray an 11" x 7" baking dish with cooking spray. Measure apple juice concentrate, flour, and orange peel into the pan, and use a whisk to stir to mix. Add sliced apples and cranberries, and toss to coat. Sprinkle with granola. Bake for 40 minutes or until the apples are tender.

174 calories per serving
0 fat, 2 gm. protein, 42 gm. carbohydrate,
0 cholesterol, 27 mg. sodium.

For exchange diets, count: 1 starch, 1 1/2 fruit.

Cranberry Soufflé

Preparation time: 15 minutes
Chilling time: at least 2 hours

12 servings—1 square each

1 pound fresh cranberries
8-ounce can crushed pineapple, drained and juice saved
3-ounce package sugar-free raspberry gelatin
2 cups nonfat sugar-free vanilla yogurt
garnish: fresh orange slices

1. Place cranberries in a saucepan. Add drained pineapple juice to the berries. Cook cranberries over medium heat for 10 minutes, until cranberries begin to soften and pop open. Stir in gelatin, and remove from the heat. Fold in yogurt. Transfer to an 11" x 7" baking pan.

2. Chill for at least 2 hours and then cut into 12 squares and serve on dessert plates. Garnish with orange slices.

36 calories per serving
0 fat, 2 gm. protein, 7 gm. carbohydrate,
0 cholesterol, 30 mg. sodium.

For exchange diets, count: 1/2 starch.

Creamy Blueberry Soup

Preparation time: 10 minutes
Chilling time: 1 hour

8 servings—2/3 cup each

2 pints fresh blueberries, washed and stemmed (may substitute
   raspberries or strawberries)
1/2 cup Equal Measure sugar substitute
1/4 cup red wine
1 teaspoon finely grated lemon rind
1 cup reduced-fat sour cream

1. Combine fresh blueberries, sugar substitute, and red wine in a
2-quart bowl. Stir for 5 minutes to fully dissolve the sugar substitute
and allow flavors to blend. Fold in lemon rind and sour cream. Chill for
at least an hour or until serving time.

76 calories per serving
0 fat, 3 gm. protein, 16 gm. carbohydrate,
1 mg. cholesterol, 45 mg. sodium.

For exchange diets, count: 1 starch.

Creamy Cherry Pie

Preparation time: 20 minutes
Chilling time: 2 hours

8 servings—1 slice each

8 ounces reduced-fat cream cheese softened
1/2 cup Equal Measure sugar substitute
1 teaspoon almond extract
reduced-fat prepared graham cracker crust
1 cup nonfat vanilla yogurt
24-ounce can sugar-free cherry pie filling

1. Beat softened cream cheese with sugar substitute in a mixing bowl with an electric mixer. Add almond extract, and beat again. Fold in yogurt, then spread in the prepared crust.

2. Spread pie filling over the cheese layer, and refrigerate at least 2 hours.

235 calories per serving
3 gm. fat, 6 gm. protein, 44 gm. carbohydrate,
2 mg. cholesterol, 288 mg. sodium.

For exchange diets, count: 2 starch, 1 fruit.

Date Bars

Preparation time: 15 minutes
Baking time: 25 minutes

12 servings—1/12 pan each

nonstick cooking spray
1 cup golden raisins
1 large baking apple, peeled and chopped fine
1/2 cup chopped dates
1 cup apple juice, divided
1/4 cup vegetable oil
2 eggs, beaten, or 1/2 cup liquid egg substitute
1 teaspoon vanilla
1 cup flour
1 teaspoon baking soda

1. Preheat oven to 350°.

2. Spray a 9-inch square baking pan with cooking spray.

3. In a large saucepan, cook raisins, apples, and dates in 1/2 cup apple juice over medium heat for 3 minutes. Remove from heat. Stir in remaining 1/2 cup apple juice, oil, beaten eggs, and vanilla. Fold in flour and soda. Spread dough into prepared pan, and bake for 25 minutes.

170 calories per serving
5 gm. fat, 3 gm. protein, 30 gm. carbohydrate,
0 cholesterol with egg substitute
(29 mg. cholesterol with egg), 126 mg. sodium.

For exchange diets, count: 1 fruit, 1 starch, 1/2 fat.

Elegant Broiled Pineapple

Preparation time: 15 minutes
Broiling time: 8 minutes

4 servings—2 slices each

1 large fresh pineapple, or one can pineapple rings, drained
2 tablespoons sweet white wine
1 tablespoon finely grated orange rind
2 tablespoons chopped pecans

1. If using fresh pineapple, cut off pineapple crown and stem end with sharp knife. Cut crosswise into 8 slices. Cut off peel; remove eyes and core.

2. Place pineapple slices on a baking sheet. Sprinkle pineapple with white wine, grated orange rind, and chopped pecans. Broil for 8 minutes under low heat.

74 calories per serving
5 gm. fat, 4 gm. protein, 7 gm. carbohydrate,
0 cholesterol, 1 mg. sodium.

For exchange diets, count: 1 fat, 1/2 fruit.

Everyone's Favorite Strawberry Pie

If you don't like a pretzel crust, use a reduced-fat graham cracker crust.

Preparation time: 20 minutes
Baking time: 20 minutes
Chilling time: 4 hours

12 servings—1 slice each

Pretzel crust:
  1 cup crushed pretzels
  2 tablespoons soft margarine
  1/2 cup nonfat sour cream
  1/2 cup flour

Filling:
  1 quart fresh strawberries
  1 cup water
  3 tablespoons apple juice concentrate
  3 tablespoons cornstarch
  1/4 cup sugar-free strawberry flavored gelatin

Topping:
  1 cup reduced-fat whipped topping

1. Preheat oven to 350°.

2. Crush pretzels in a blender container to make 1 cup coarse crumbs.

3. Combine pretzel crumbs with margarine, sour cream, and flour in a mixing bowl. Press pretzel mixture into a 9" pie plate, using your fingers to spread evenly. Bake for 20 minutes.

4. When crust is done, clean and stem berries, and slice into the crust.

5. Combine water, apple juice concentrate, and cornstarch in a small saucepan. Bring mixture to boil, stirring constantly. Boil for 2 minutes. Stir in sugar-free gelatin. Pour over berries. Refrigerate for at least 2 hours.

6. Garnish each slice with 3 tablespoons reduced-fat whipped topping.

200 calories per serving
5 gm. fat, 3 gm. protein, 40 gm. carbohydrate,
0 cholesterol, 418 mg. sodium.

For exchange diets, count: 2 starch, 1/2 fruit.

Frozen Fruit Cups

Preparation time: 15 minutes
Freezing time: 6 hours

16 servings—2/3 cup each

16-ounce bag frozen whole strawberries
20-ounce can crushed pineapple in juice
20-ounce can apricots in juice, quartered
4 fresh bananas, peeled and sliced 1/4-inch thick
12-ounce can sugar-free lemon lime soft drink

Garnish:
1 cup nonfat sour cream
1/2 teaspoon vanilla
1 teaspoon Nutrasweet Spoonful sugar substitute

1. Combine fruits, their juices, and the soft drink in a large bowl. Stir to mix, then ladle into muffin cups. Freeze for 6 hours.

2. Meanwhile, combine sour cream with vanilla and sugar substitute in a small bowl; cover. To remove frozen fruit cups from the muffin tin, dip bottom of muffin tin in a shallow pan of very hot water. Gently remove the fruit cups with a spoon. Place them in a fruit dish, and garnish with sour cream mixture.

105 calories per serving
0 fat, 1 gm. protein, 23 gm. carbohydrate,
0 cholesterol, 24 mg. sodium.

For exchange diets, count: 1 1/2 fruit.

Kahlua Mousse

Preparation time: 15 minutes
Chilling time: 2 hours

8 servings—1/2 cup each

1/3 cup Kahlua Café instant coffee beverage
2 tablespoons hot water
2 1/2 cups skim milk
1 package (6 servings) chocolate flavor fat-free, sugar-free
   instant pudding mix
1 cup reduced-fat whipped topping, softened

1. Dissolve instant coffee in water in a medium mixing bowl. Pour milk into the coffee mixture, and stir to mix. Whisk in pudding mix, and beat for 2 minutes. Fold in whipped topping and spoon into 8 dessert dishes. Chill for at least 2 hours or until ready to serve.

110 calories per serving
3 gm. fat, 3 gm. protein, 17 gm. carbohydrate,
0 cholesterol, 290 mg. sodium.

For exchange diets, count: 1 starch, 1/2 fat.

Kiwi Frozen Fruit Treats

Preparation time: 15 minutes
Freezing time: 3 hours

8 servings—5 ounces each

4 large, firm kiwifruit
6-ounce can pineapple juice concentrate
2 cups sugar-free lemon lime-soft drink

1. Peel kiwifruit and process in a blender just until smooth; do not crush the seeds. Stir in pineapple juice concentrate and soft drink. Pour mixture into 8 (6-ounce) paper cups. Freeze at least 3 hours.

2. To eat, remove cups from freezer, microwave for 30 seconds on high power, and then eat as a slush with a spoon.

34 calories per serving
0 fat, 0 protein, 8 gm. carbohydrate,
0 cholesterol, 11 mg. sodium.

For exchange diets, count: 1/2 fruit.

Lemon Angel Cookies

Preparation time: 20 minutes
Baking time: 12 minutes

48 servings—1 cookie each

nonstick cooking spray
1/2 cup margarine, softened
1 1/4 cups sugar or 1 1/4 cup Sugar Twin Spoonable sugar substitute
1/2 cup nonfat sugar-free lemon yogurt
1 egg
1 tablespoon grated lemon peel
1/2 teaspoon vanilla
2 cups quick oats
1 1/2 cups flour
1 teaspoon baking powder
1/2 teaspoon baking soda

1. Preheat oven to 350°.

2. Spray a baking sheet with cooking spray.

3. In a large mixing bowl, beat margarine and sugar until creamy. Add yogurt, egg, lemon peel, and vanilla, and beat well. Add all remaining ingredients, and mix well.

4. With lightly floured hands, form 1-inch balls from the dough. Use a glass dipped in flour to flatten each cookie. Bake for 12 minutes or until the edges are light brown. Cool for 2 minutes before removing to a wire rack.

51 calories per serving (31 calories with sugar substitute)
1 gm. fat, 0 protein, 10 gm. carbohydrate (4 gm. carbohydrate with sugar substitute), 5 mg. cholesterol, 32 mg. sodium.

For exchange diets, count: 1/2 starch.

Lemon Cheesecake in a Reduced-Fat Crust

Preparation time: 15 minutes
Baking time: 40 minutes

8 servings—1 slice each

Filling:
>   2 cups fat-free ricotta cheese
>   1/2 cup Sugar Twin Spoonable sugar substitute
>   1/3 cup skim milk
>   2 tablespoons flour
>   2 tablespoons fresh squeezed lemon juice
>   1 tablespoon finely grated lemon peel
>   1 teaspoon vanilla
>   1/4 teaspoon salt
>   2 eggs or 1/2 cup liquid egg substitute

Reduced-fat prepared graham cracker crust

1. Preheat oven to 350°.

2. Combine ingredients for the filling in a mixing bowl, and beat with an electric mixer until smooth. Pour filling into the crust. Bake for 40 minutes or until the center of the cheesecake is almost set. Cool to room temperature, then store in the refrigerator.

165 calories per serving
4 gm. fat, 12 gm. protein, 23 gm. carbohydrate,
43 mg. cholesterol (6 mg. cholesterol with
egg substitute), 268 mg. sodium.

For exchange diets, count: 1 skim milk, 1 starch.

Minted Honeydew Melon

Preparation time: 15 minutes
Chilling time: 30 minutes to 24 hours

8 servings—1 1/2 cup each

2 medium honeydew melons
1/4 cup white crème de menthe
1/2 cup white wine
1 teaspoon poppy seeds

1. Remove rinds from melons, scoop out seeds, and form balls from the flesh.

2. Combine crème de menthe, wine cooler, and poppy seeds in a large salad bowl. Add melon balls to the mint marinade, cover and refrigerate at least 30 minutes or up to 24 hours before serving.

3. Use a slotted spoon to serve the melon into a fruit bowl.

83 calories per serving
0 fat, 1 gm. protein, 20 gm. carbohydrate,
0 cholesterol, 22 mg. sodium.

For exchange diets, count: 1 1/2 fruit.

Oatmeal Raisin Cookies

Go ahead and refrigerate half of this dough for fresh cookies next week.

Preparation time: 20 minutes
Baking time: 12 minutes per baking sheet
36 servings—1 cookie each

1/3 cup brown sugar, or Sugar Twin brown sugar substitute
1/4 cup apple juice concentrate
2/3 cup soft margarine
2 eggs or 1/2 cup liquid egg substitute
1 teaspoon baking soda
1/2 teaspoon salt
1/2 teaspoon cinnamon
1 teaspoon vanilla
1/2 teaspoon nutmeg
1 1/2 cups flour
1 1/2 cups quick oats
2/3 cup raisins

1. Preheat oven to 350°.

2. In a large mixing bowl, beat brown sugar or substitute, apple juice concentrate, and margarine until creamy. Add eggs and mix well.

3. In a separate bowl, mix soda, salt, cinnamon, vanilla, and nutmeg together. Add it to the creamed mixture, and blend. Fold in flour, oats, and raisins.

4. Drop by spoonfuls on a nonstick baking sheet, and bake for about 12 minutes.

60 calories per serving (53 calories with sugar substitute)
2 gm. fat, 1 gm. protein, 10 gm. carbohydrate
(8 gm. carbohydrate with sugar substitute), 12 mg. cholesterol
(0 cholesterol with egg substitute), 94 mg. sodium.

For exchange diets, count: 1 fruit.

Peach Pie in a Shortbread Crust

Preparation time: 20 minutes
Baking time: 40 minutes

8 servings—1 slice each

1 prepared shortbread crust (such as Keebler)
6 large ripe peaches (or nectarines)
2 tablespoons flour
1 teaspoon nutmeg
1/4 teaspoon salt
1 cup evaporated skim milk
1 cup low-fat granola

1. Preheat oven to 350°.

2. Peel and thinly slice peaches into the prepared crust. In a small bowl, mix flour, nutmeg, and salt together. Sprinkle over the peaches, and toss to mix. Pour milk over the peaches, and top with granola. Bake for 40 minutes.

248 calories per serving
3 gm. fat, 6 gm. protein, 49 gm. carbohydrate,
0 cholesterol, 224 mg. sodium.

For exchange diets, count: 1 1/2 starch, 1 1/2 fruit, 1/2 skim milk.

Peppermint Pears

Preparation time: 20 minutes
Chilling time: 2 hours

4 servings—1 cup each

1 1/2 cups evaporated skim milk
2 whole eggs, well beaten, or 1/2 cup liquid egg substitute
1/3 cup Equal Measure sugar substitute
dash of salt
1/4 teaspoon peppermint flavor
16-ounce can pear halves in juice, drained
garnish: fresh mint leaves

1. Combine evaporated milk and beaten eggs in a saucepan. Use a whisk to stir and cook over medium heat until thickened, about 5 to 7 minutes. Pour into a bowl, and stir in sugar substitute, salt, and peppermint flavor. Chill for at least 2 hours or until serving time.

2. Divide drained pear halves among four dessert dishes. Pour peppermint sauce over the pears, and serve. Garnish with mint leaves.

155 calories per serving
1 gm. fat, 11 gm. protein, 26 gm. carbohydrate,
3 mg. cholesterol with egg substitute
(89 mg. cholesterol with egg), 159 mg. sodium.

For exchange diets, count: 1 fruit, 1 skim milk.

Pumpkin Custard

Angie Lindenberg shared this idea with me.

Preparation time: 20 minutes
Baking time: 45 minutes

12 servings—1 square each

16-ounce can solid pumpkin
13-ounce can evaporated skim milk
1/4 cup liquid egg substitute
1/2 cup reduced-fat baking mix
2 tablespoons sugar
4 packages Sweet One sweetener
2 teaspoons pumpkin pie spice
2 teaspoons vanilla
nonstick cooking spray

1. Preheat oven to 350°.

2. In a large mixing bowl, combine all ingredients, then beat smooth with an electric mixer. Pour into an 11" x 7" baking dish that has been sprayed with cooking spray. Bake for 45 minutes or until mixture is set.

77 calories per serving
0 fat, 4 gm. protein, 12 gm. carbohydrate,
1 mg. cholesterol, 139 mg. sodium.

For exchange diets, count: 1 starch.

Raspberry Cream Cheese Pie

Preparation time: 20 minutes
Chilling time: 2 hours

8 servings—1 slice each

8 ounces reduced-fat cream cheese
1/2 cup all-fruit raspberry preserves
8 ounces sugar-free raspberry yogurt
reduced-fat graham cracker pie crust
2 cups fresh raspberries
1/3 cup all-fruit raspberry preserves
1 teaspoon almond extract

1. In a medium mixing bowl, beat cream cheese and 1/2 cup preserves with an electric mixer on medium speed until smooth. Fold in yogurt, then spread into the prepared pie crust.

2. Spread fresh raspberries over the top.

3. In a glass measuring cup, warm 1/3 cup raspberry preserves in microwave for 1 minute on high power. Stir in almond extract, and drizzle preserves over the berries. Cover and chill at least 2 hours or until serving.

243 calories per serving
4 gm. fat, 6 gm. protein, 45 gm. carbohydrate,
2 mg. cholesterol, 270 mg. sodium.

For exchange diets, count: 2 starch, 1 fruit, 1/2 fat.

Rum and Raisin Bread Pudding

Preparation time: 15 minutes
Baking time: 40 minutes

16 servings—1/16 pan each

4 eggs or 1 cup liquid egg substitute
1 1/2 cups apple juice concentrate
1 tablespoon rum extract
1 tablespoon cinnamon
1 tablespoon nutmeg
1 tablespoon vanilla
2 tablespoons margarine, melted
3 cups skim milk
nonstick cooking spray
6 cups bread cubes
1/2 cup coconut
1/2 cup raisins

1. Preheat oven to 375°.

2. In a mixing bowl, beat first 8 ingredients until smooth.

3. Spray an 11" x 7" baking dish with cooking spray. Layer bread cubes, coconut, and raisins in the dish. Pour egg and milk mixture over bread. Bake for 40 minutes or until set. Allow bread pudding to cool slightly, then cut and serve.

243 calories per serving
5 gm. fat, 8 gm. protein, 40 gm. carbohydrate,
54 mg. cholesterol (0 cholesterol with egg substitute),
408 mg. sodium.

For exchange diets, count: 1 fruit, 2 starch, 1/2 fat.

Strawberry Dessert Soufflé

Preparation time: 20 minutes
Chilling time: 2 1/2 hours

8 servings—3/4 cup each

2 (3-ounce) packages sugar-free strawberry gelatin
1 cup boiling water
1 cup sugar-free lemon-lime soft drink
3 ounces nonfat cream cheese, softened
1/4 cup reduced-fat mayonnaise
1 quart fresh strawberries
1/4 cup chopped pecans

1. In a mixing bowl, combine gelatin with boiling water, stirring to completely dissolve gelatin. Add soft drink, and stir again. Add softened cream cheese and mayonnaise, and use a whisk to stir until smooth. Refrigerate this for 30 minutes.

2. Wash strawberries, and use a food chopper to chop fine. Remove gelatin from refrigerator and fold in chopped berries. Turn mixture into a soufflé dish, and garnish with nuts. Refrigerate until firm or about 2 hours. Loosen the soufflé by gently dipping the dish in a shallow pan of warm water. Slice, and serve on dessert plates.

95 calories per serving
5 gm. fat, 2 gm. protein, 12 gm. carbohydrate,
1 mg. cholesterol, 135 mg. sodium.

For exchange diets, count: 1 fruit, 1 fat.

Strawberry Shortcake

Preparation time: 20 minutes
Baking time: 10 minutes

12 servings—1 cake + 1/3 cup berries each

2 1/2 cups reduced-fat baking mix
3 tablespoons soft margarine, melted
1/2 cup fat-free sugar-free vanilla yogurt
4 cups fresh strawberries, washed, stemmed, and sliced
1/4 cup Equal Measure sugar substitute
garnish: dollop of fat-free sugar-free vanilla yogurt

1. Preheat oven to 450°.

2. Mix baking mix, margarine, and yogurt in a mixing bowl until a soft dough forms. Gently smooth the dough into a ball on a floured surface. Knead the dough 8 times. Roll the dough out to about 1/2-inch thick. Cut out 12 cakes with a floured 3-inch round cutter.

3. Place shortcakes on an ungreased baking sheet, and bake for 10 minutes. Remove from the oven, and cool.

4. Meanwhile, combine sliced berries with sugar substitute in a bowl, and chill.

5. Cut shortcakes in half, place both halves on a dessert plate, and spoon berries on top. Garnish with yogurt if desired.

172 calories per serving
4 gm. fat, 4 gm. protein, 30 gm. carbohydrate,
0 cholesterol, 500 mg. sodium.

For exchange diets, count: 1 fruit, 1 starch, 1 fat.

Sugar-Free Spiced Fruit

Preparation time: 15 minutes
Chilling time: 30 minutes

16 servings—3/4 cup each

1 fresh pineapple
3 fresh peaches
3 fresh pears
1 pound seedless green grapes
1 cup apple juice concentrate
thin peelings from 1 orange
1/4 cup orange juice
3 cinnamon sticks
6 whole allspice

1. Remove crown from pineapple and discard. Peel pineapple, and cut into wedges, discarding center core. Cut into 1-inch chunks. Place in a large glass or plastic bowl with a tight-fitting cover.

2. Core the peaches and pears and cut into chunks. Add to the pineapple. Remove stems from grapes, and add to fruit mixture.

3. In a small saucepan, combine all remaining ingredients. Boil for 3 minutes. Pour over fruit. Mix well, cover, and refrigerate for at least 30 minutes. This tasty fruit salad keeps in the refrigerator for 5 days.

88 calories per serving
0 fat, 1 gm. protein, 22 gm. carbohydrate,
0 cholesterol, 1 mg. sodium.

For exchange diets, count: 1 1/2 fruit.

Unforgettable Aloha Dessert

Preparation time: 20 minutes
Chilling time: at least 3 hours

12 servings—1 square each

nonstick cooking spray
1 1/2 cups graham cracker crumbs
2 tablespoons soft margarine, melted
20-ounce can crushed pineapple, undrained
3 tablespoons flour
3-ounce package sugar-free orange gelatin
16-ounce can dark sweet cherries, drained
5 small bananas, diced
1/2 cup NutraSweet Equal Measure sugar substitute

Toppings:
    1 cup reduced-fat whipped topping
    2 tablespoons chopped pecans
    2 tablespoons shredded coconut

1. Preheat oven to 375°.

2. Spray an 11" x 7" baking dish with cooking spray. Combine melted margarine and graham cracker crumbs in the dish; pat the mixture firmly over the bottom on the dish. Bake for 15 minutes.

3. Meanwhile, in a saucepan, mix pineapple and flour together. Bring the mixture to a boil, stirring occasionally with a whisk. Remove from the heat, and add the gelatin. Cool for 15 minutes, then fold in drained cherries, bananas, and sugar substitute. Pour over the crust.

4. Spread whipped topping over the gelatin and fruit layer, sprinkle with pecans and coconut, and chill for 3 hours or until the dessert is firm.

257 calories per serving
5 gm. fat, 4 gm. protein, 53 gm. carbohydrate,
0 cholesterol, 195 mg. sodium.

For exchange diets, count: 2 starch, 1 1/2 fruit.

Appendices
and
Index

The Language of Diabetes

As you use this book, you may have been talking about glucose and cholesterol levels for a long time. But for the benefit of readers less comfortable with all the terms, let's review some common words used in the book.

blood glucose level—the concentration of glucose in the blood, normally expressed as the weight (milligrams) of glucose found in 100 milliliters (about 1/3 cup) of blood. Normal levels are generally between 80 and 125 mg/100 ml. This is often expressed as mg/dl.

blood glucose monitoring—measuring blood glucose levels from a blood sample taken from a finger prick, involving the use of a home-based hand-held blood glucose monitor.

carbohydrate—one of the three major energy sources in foods, and includes sugars and starches (4 calories per gram).

cholesterol—a fat-like substance normally found in blood shown to be a major factor in developing heart disease.

exchange—foods grouped together on a list according to similarities in food values.

fat—one of the three major energy sources in food (9 calories per gram).

fiber—an indigestible part of food, also known as roughage and bulk.

glucose—a single unit of carbohydrate energy; the final breakdown product of sugars and starches that is absorbed through the stomach or intestinal wall into the blood. Requires insulin for transport out of the blood.

insulin—a hormone made by the body that helps the body use

food by carrying glucose out of the blood and to the cells where it can be used for energy.

insulin-dependent diabetes mellitus (IDDM)—the type of diabetes that is managed by insulin injections together with diet, more common in young people.

non-insulin dependent diabetes (NIDDM)—the type of diabetes that is managed by medicines together with diet, more common in older overweight people.

polyunsaturated and monounsaturated fat—These types of fats are usually liquid at room temperature. These are the fats of choice to lower high blood cholesterol when used as part of a low-fat, high-fiber diet.

saturated fat—the type of fat that tends to raise blood cholesterol levels. It comes primarily from animal foods and is usually stiff at room temperature.

triglycerides—fat normally present in the blood, made from food. Weight gain, a high-fat diet, and alcohol or sugar intake may increase blood triglycerides.

Resources

Look to these organizations for additional help in answering your questions about managing diabetes.

American Diabetes Association
1990 Duke Street
Alexandria, VA 22314
1-800-232-3472

Recently the American Diabetes Association kicked off a campaign to get the word out that black Americans are twice as likely as others to develop diabetes. For the past 30 years, there has been a steady increase in the number of African Americans who are diagnosed with the disease. The American Diabetes Association estimates that 2.6 million African Americans, including 1 out of every 4 black women over the age of 55, have diabetes. Order *Diabetes Forecast* monthly magazine from this group.

American Dietetic Association
National Center for Nutrition and Dietetics
216 West Jackson Boulevard
Chicago, IL 60606
1-800-366-1655

Talk with a registered dietitian, or order the *Exchange Lists* and other written materials from the group that represents almost 70,000 diet and nutrition professionals in the United States.

Juvenile Diabetes Foundation International
432 Park Avenue South
New York, NY 10157-0706
1-800-223-1138

Contact this organization to become actively involved in raising funds for diabetes research.

Diabetes Self-Management
PO Box 52890
Boulder, CO 80322-2890
This magazine is printed every other month.

References

American Dietetic Association. "Nutrition recommendations and principles for people with diabetes mellitus." *Journal of the American Dietetic Association.* May, 1994, page 504.

American Dietetic Association. "Position on the use of nutritive and nonnutritive sweeteners." *Journal of the American Dietetic Association.* July, 1993, page 816.

American Dietetic Association. *Enhancing food flavor with herbs and spices.* Chicago, IL: The American Dietetic Association, 1995.

American Dietetic Association. *Meal Planning Approaches for Diabetes Management.* Chicago, IL: The American Dietetic Association, 1995.

Anthan, George. "Food concerns rooted in psyche, study says." *Des Moines Register,* January 25, 1996, page 1.

Carper, Jean. "The spices of life." *USA Weekend.* February 2, 1996, page 20.

Cavaiani, Mabel. *The New Diabetic Cookbook.* Chicago, IL: Contemporary Books, 1994, pages 74-81.

Exchange Lists for Meal Planning. Chicago, IL: American Diabetes Association and American Dietetic Association, 1995.

Franz, Marion, "Nutritional strategies for diabetes control." *RD,* Fall, 1995. page 3.

Levy, Doug. "Spreading word to blacks about diabetes risk." *USA Today.* February 5, 1996, page 1.

Milchovich, Sue. *Diabetes Mellitus.* Palo Alto: Bull Publishing Co. 1992.

Oster, Gerry. "Estimated effects of reducing dietary saturated fat intake on the incidence and costs of coronary heart disease in the United States." *Journal of the American Dietetic Association.* February, 1996, page 127.

Sanders, Bonnie. *Joslin Diabetes Gourmet Cookbook.* New York: Bantam Books, page 446, 1995.

What's This Stuff? A Parent's Guide To Coping with Picky Eaters. Lakeville-Middleboro, Massachusetts: Ocean Spray Cranberries, Inc. 1995.

Index